Praise for Stephanie Marango, Rebecca Gordon, and

Your Body
and the Stars

"Rebecca Gordon is one of the best astrologers I've ever met. She's authentic, funny, and extremely talented! I recommend her work and *Your Body and the Stars* to everyone!"
—**Gabby Bernstein**, *New York Times* bestselling author of *Miracles Now*

"I love how Dr. Stephanie and Rebecca take your body and soul to another dimension with merging the physical, metaphysical, and mind with in-depth exploration of relating ourselves to every zodiac sign. *Your Body and the Stars* deeply educated me on opening my eyes on how much I needed to use elements of the other signs to make me whole. Brilliant!"
—**Elisabeth Halfpapp**, executive vice president of Mind-body Programming, cofounder of exhale, cocreator of Core Fusion™ barre, and coauthor of *Barre Fitness*

"This is a beautiful book by Dr. Stephanie and Rebecca Gordon. I have been fascinated with astrology and health for nearly fifty years and what these women have put together is informative and helpful for anyone interested in astrology and body relationships, and how you can use them for greater well-being. I highly recommend *Your Body and the Stars*."
—**Elson M. Haas, MD**, integrative family physician (elsonhaasmd.com) and author of *Staying Healthy with the Seasons* and *Staying Healthy with Nutrition*

"Carl Sagan said, 'We are made of star-stuff,' and in their groundbreaking new book, *Your Body and the Stars*, astrologer Rebecca Gordon and holistic physician Dr. Stephanie back up this powerful cosmic concept with an integrative wellness guide that shows you, through practical tools and a cosmically artful health program, how to maximize your overall well-being. Through understanding the relationship between the signs and your physical body, Rebecca and Dr. Stephanie take you on a journey of self-discovery that will bring you into harmony with the stars and the physical world and show you how to live in optimal wellness."

—**Ronnie Grishman**, editor-in-chief, *Dell Horoscope* magazine

"Bravo, Dr. Stephanie and Rebecca! I am now fascinated to know that my physical body, and all that I ask it to do, is so profoundly influenced by my metaphysical connection to the universe. The wisdom that I have taken from these pages has deepened my appreciation of my body and my understanding of the Mind-Body concept, which is so prevalent in our fitness programs at exhale. Thanks for such a great read. This will now be one of my reference books!"

—**Fred DeVito**, executive vice president and cofounder of exhale, cocreator of Core Fusion™ barre, and coauthor of *Barre Fitness*

Your Body and the Stars

THE ZODIAC AS YOUR WELLNESS GUIDE

STEPHANIE MARANGO, MD, RYT
and REBECCA GORDON

ATRIA PAPERBACK
New York London Toronto Sydney New Delhi

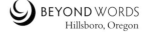
BEYOND WORDS
Hillsboro, Oregon

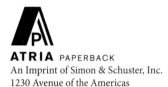

ATRIA PAPERBACK
An Imprint of Simon & Schuster, Inc.
1230 Avenue of the Americas
New York, NY 10020

BEYOND WORDS
20827 N.W. Cornell Road, Suite 500
Hillsboro, Oregon 97124-9808
503-531-8700 / 503-531-8773 fax
www.beyondword.com

Managing editor: Lindsay S. Easterbrooks-Brown
Editors: Emmalisa Sparrow, Emily Han, Gretchen Stelter
Copyeditor: Ali McCart
Proofreader: Jenefer Angell
Cover design: Devon Smith
Composition: William H. Brunson Typography Services

First Atria Paperback/Beyond Words trade paperback edition May 2016

ATRIA PAPERBACK and colophon are trademarks of Simon & Schuster, Inc.

Beyond Words Publishing is an imprint of Simon & Schuster, Inc., and the Beyond Words logo is a registered trademark of Beyond Words Publishing, Inc.

For more information about special discounts for bulk purchases, please contact Simon & Schuster Special Sales at 1-866-506-1949 or business@simonandschuster.com.

The Simon & Schuster Speakers Bureau can bring authors to your live event. For more information or to book an event, contact the Simon & Schuster Speakers Bureau at 1-866-248-3049 or visit our website at www.simonspeakers.com.

Manufactured in the United States of America

10 9 8 7 6 5 4 3 2 1

Library of Congress Cataloging-in-Publication Data

Names: Marango, Stephanie P., author.
Title: Your body and the stars : the zodiac as your wellness guide/Stephanie P. Marango, MD, RYT and Rebecca Gordon.
Description: First Atria Paperback/Beyond Words trade paperback edition. Hillsboro, Oregon : Beyond Words, 2016. | Includes bibliographical references and index.
Identifiers: LCCN 2015040665 (print) | LCCN 2015043631 (ebook) | ISBN 9781582704906 (pbk. : alk. paper) | ISBN 9781476771472 (eBook)
Subjects: LCSH: Astrology and health. | Zodiac. | Human body—Miscellanea. Classification: LCC BF1729.H9 M37 2016 (print) | LCC BF1729.H9 (ebook) | DDC 133.5/861—dc23
LC record available at http://lccn.loc.gov/2015040665

ISBN 978-1-58270-490-6
ISBN 978-1-4767-7147-2 (ebook)

The corporate mission of Beyond Words Publishing, Inc.: *Inspire to Integrity*

Contents

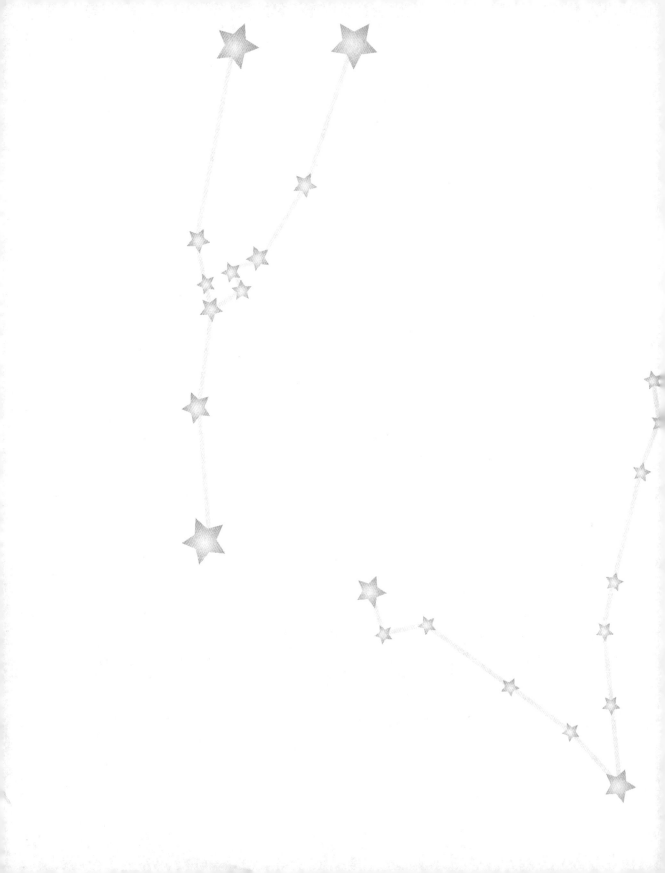

Preface

As a believer in both science and spirituality, I know that energy takes myriad forms. In fact, I see science and spirituality as often saying similar things, just in different ways. But the science books and I diverge: I don't limit myself exclusively to them—to accepting as possible only what our current technologies can perceive. Just as ultraviolet rays and microorganisms existed well before we developed the proper tools to see them, I believe that there is still so much more out there than meets our modern eyes and minds. Who am I to limit nature's abilities—or our means of understanding them?

This is the mind-set with which I greeted Rebecca's astrology presentation during a conference on the evolution of consciousness in 2012. Previously, I had never thought much about astrology. Sure, I knew my sun (birth) sign (Sagittarius) and had flipped through some horoscopes, but beyond basic pop culture it had not substantially entered my purview. So I was surprised that her talk had such an impact on me. But it did! And I believe it did because Rebecca explained the stars in the same vein that I understand—in my work as a holistic physician—the human body: as practical magic.

In my definition, *practical magic* is the ability to take unseen forces in our world—like thoughts, emotions, sensations, intuitions, and beyond—and embody them; it is giving the formless form. Like how a thought in your head—such as, *I want to buy a house*—one day translates into something tangible—an actual brick-and-mortar dwelling that you and the rest of your material belongings occupy; or how unresolved emotional stress with your boss at work becomes tension in the muscles of your neck. In my mind, that's a kind of magic.

And it's practical because it pertains to your everyday life. Your thoughts, feelings, and impressions are ultimately expressed in what you choose to eat, how you choose to spend your time, with whom you choose to spend it, etc. You are the magician who gets to choose both the formless and its form! Sometimes, your choices on the outside reflect your true nature on the inside, but that's not always the case. You might not always feel congruent or balanced in how you are living—which creates a sense of dis-ease. Your fullest expression of health is nothing less than your fullest expression of self.

Which leads us to back to Rebecca and her ability to read your birth chart to glean the cosmos within. Whether her client is a stay-at-home mom or a corporate professional, Rebecca reminds everyone of what makes them unique, from the pattern of their fingerprints to the blueprint of their soul. Reading their stars to align them with their greater wisdom, she motivates them to move outside of their comfort zones, to live the most expansive versions of their lives.

For example, she might guide a client who is a Taurus to broaden his self-expression, which will not only help him align with his true nature but also help resolve tension in his neck. I, similarly, would empower a patient who has chronic neck tension with a greater understanding of her body and its connection to her mind, emotions, and spirit; how her intangible thoughts, feelings, and stories around self-expression (which is represented both physically and metaphysically by the neck) may result in tangible muscle tension and stress. And then I would teach her practical tools—movement, breath, nutrition, meditation, and more—to address it.

So while Rebecca and I might outwardly seem like an unorthodox pair (or the beginning of a joke about a doctor and an astrologer walking into a bar . . .), we both approach our personal and professional lives with the ingrained belief that everything is within, that your body contains a universe of wisdom that may serve as a key to your well-being—if you let it.

Of course, we weren't aware of this conceptual overlap until we met, which didn't happen that evening at the conference. Yes, that first night I saw her, I just knew that we were going to meet one day and have a profound relationship. But it needed to happen at the right time. And so I just sat and smiled during her talk, woke up the next day inspired to outline this book . . . and then waited about six months until it turned out that the office space I was renting in a healing center was directly next to hers. Talk about our stars aligning!

And the rest is, well, this book. A book about your body and the stars. A fresh perspective that allows you to awaken and rise to new possibilities, beyond the constraints of who you currently imagine you are or should be . . . along with practical tools to help you live the fullest, richest, most well life possible. Isn't it time for you to reclaim your full self? To be your own expert on you? If so, if you feel that for as happy and healthy as you are, there is still more—and you want to take hands-on responsibility for it—then we invite you to explore this next chapter of your story. A story of heaven and earth, spirit and matter, and you, the individual who resides in between.

—Dr. Stephanie

Introduction

This is not an astrology book, nor an anatomy one. Rather, it is a wellness guide, one that uses the stars as its foundation versus a specific diet or exercise routine. There are many ways to be healthy and feel well. And fortunately, our contemporary focus is beginning to shift toward holistic wellness as a new model of health. Make no mistake—we believe the traditional Western medical system, while it has its flaws, does a good job. But it focuses on acute care and disease diagnosis and management—not health optimization and wellness.

Wellness is more encompassing. It is not just of the body, but also of the mind, emotions, and spirit. When we enter into these intangible realms, though, many wellness modalities become hard to prove with our current scientific yardsticks and measures—after all, assessing one's emotional or mental well-being is more nebulous than examining X-rays for broken bones. But one reason holistic modalities are now more mainstream than alternative is that most people who experience nutrition, yoga, acupuncture, and the like do not require any further proof than the way they feel. For most of us, the proof is in our personal health, experience, and understanding.

This book presents another way to access all your tangible and intangible bits and pieces, and to help them start functioning as a unified whole. On first glimpse, a methodology that uses the zodiac for wellness may seem a bit out there, but we're just reclaiming an ancient and acknowl-edged belief system—one that is an underpinning of modern medicine and science, regardless of any misconceptions or controversy. As the scientific historian Dr. David Lindberg reminds us, "If we wish to do justice to the historical enterprise, we must take the past for what it was. . . . We must respect the way earlier generations approached nature, acknowledging that although it may differ from the modern way, it is nonethe-less of interest because it is part of our intellectual ancestry."[1] So, in using this book, we are asking you to not only take increased responsibility for your well-being, but also to try a new way of doing it—one that will expand, engage, and inspire your understand-ing of health and wellness unlike before.

The story of the stars presents powerful principles that enable you to achieve your fullest expression of wellness, which is your fullest expression of self. If you put your attention toward these principles in relationship to your body, you will begin to realize that you are so much more than meets the eye. Sure, you will feel better and more comfortable in your own skin, but the true gift of the book is that it can help guide you to live the best version of yourself at *all* levels—body, mind, and spirit. In so doing, you will realize a life that is more textured—with a radiant body, inspiring thoughts, expanded emotions, and trustworthy intuition. And ulti-mately your personal microcosm will reconnect to the macrocosm to which you naturally belong.

About the Book

Your Body and the Stars uses the zodiac as a map of your physical form and, from head to feet, symbolizes your connection to the cosmos. It helps you reclaim your body and contextualize it into your greater whole and—as you do—reclaim aspects of yourself that may have been lost or forgotten. We simply bridge their healing connection.

The first chapter, "As Above, So Below," lays the foundation for the connection. We introduce the stars in context to both astrology and your body. Then each of the next twelve chapters is devoted to a specific region of the body and its associated zodiac sign, going into more informative detail regarding your body's interrela-tionship with the stars. The body region (head, chest, knees) sets the stage for each chapter, with a focus on the musculoskeletal anatomy, as the bones, joints, and mus-cles tend to be the parts that are the most relatable and easily accessed. We then connect the body to the astrological spirit or character of the zodiac sign, which is presented via the sign's theme, and we explain the theme in order to introduce its universal characteristics while highlighting its personal relevance for you.

The Lessons sections in each chapter are intended to introduce you to mind-spirit considerations that *might* accompany your body's symptoms. They are not for self-diagnosis, nor do they imply that certain dates or traits will result in certain symptoms. Rather, they outline possible connections between the zodiac signs and physical manifestations that are more complex than presented here. Again, the emphasis is on musculoskeletal manifestations (with a glimpse of some others).

To make the material not only relevant but also practical, we then offer self-study questions to help elucidate how the signs' themes currently live within you (so be honest and nonjudgmental in your observations), as well as movement recommendations to guide you in bringing the themes to physical life. The recommended exercises are practical for most levels of experience and culled from a variety of modalities: stretching and strengthening exercises, yoga, Pilates, and beyond. As we are unable to include images for every exercise, we encourage you to ask your local movement instructors or go online to find visual instructions that accompany our written ones.

These exercises are intended to address a broad audience, with modifications to help you tailor them to your level. That said, we encourage you to further modify them to the needs of your body (for example, increasing the number of repetitions, decreasing the length of a hold, using supportive yoga blocks and cushions). Please do so with diligence, self-awareness, and proper alignment, for your greatest safety. It is often easier to perform an advanced exercise improperly than a basic one properly.

You will notice that the twelve main chapters alternate in their use of gender-specific nouns and pronouns (*he* and *she*). This usage is in accordance with the polarity of the star sign discussed. *Polarities* are dualities—yin and yang, feminine and masculine, negative and positive—that represent mutual understanding. The terms are not used pejoratively and there is no relationship to gender. For instance, fire signs like Aries are considered more yang and share certain traits like action and extroversion; as it is a masculine sign, the pronoun used in the chapter is *he*. Taurus, on the other hand, is a feminine sign so the pronoun used to describe its energy is *she*. While not the norm, we have adopted this approach to help maintain the integrity of each sign.

The book concludes with appendixes that offer useful references: a chart with examples of the different manifestations related to the zodiac-body connection, a body-of-the-stars body scan, and a reference for skeletal structures and regions of the body. In writing this book we have merely introduced the vast realms of astrology and anatomy and their healing connection; the goal of these appendixes is to enable you to keep learning and experiencing on your own.

How to Use This Book

We believe that experience is the master teacher. Many readers of astrology or anatomy books tend to read only the chapter that they believe pertains to them (for example, the Virgo sun sign reads about the Virgo and the knee surgeon reads about the knee). However, we encourage you to experience every chapter of this book, because every body region and sign lives within you! You might be a Virgo by birth, but you still have the hands of the Twins (Gemini) and the heart of a Lion (Leo). Every day the different signs express themselves differently through you.

When a body region is in need of attention due to extrinsic pain or intrinsic imbalance, the sign's susceptibilities also come to the forefront; effectively, both body and sign are in need of attention and balance with the rest of you. However, you certainly do not have to wait until a part of you feels out of whack in order to read about it. In fact, we encourage you to read about different body regions in order to optimize their health if that's what you're drawn to. In other words, we encourage you to read the chapters in the order that resonates with you. In this way, the book may be used as a custom-tailored body scan and wellness reference to use time and time again.

You can begin your scan by choosing a chapter based on either its body region or its zodiac sign. Choose the region that interests you the most. Perhaps it is correlated with your sun sign, or it is an area you recently read about in a fitness magazine, or it is an area where you feel pain. For example, if you are a runner who wants to know more about your knees, flip to chapter 11, "Knees of the Seagoat." Approach the chapter with an open mind, with questions like *What are my knees, really? What role do they play in my life? What can I learn from them?* Then, flip to the body regions above and below—in this case the "Hips of the Centaur" and "Ankles of the Water Bearer"—to learn about connected body parts that may be associated with your knee pain.

This book is also about your connection to the stars, the ancient wisdom they represent, and how you can harness their wisdom through your physical form. So you can also choose to begin with a chapter based on your sun (birth), moon, or rising sign, or on one of the signs' themes that you wish to further embody. For example, if you are a Pisces sun sign who wants to know more about your nature and how to best express it, turn to chapter 13, "Feet of the Fish." While reading, ask questions like

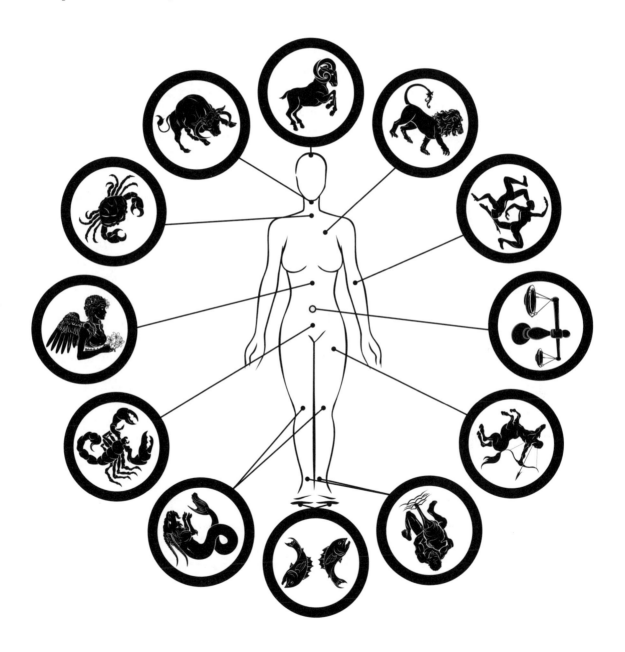

How do I live the nature of the Fish? What lessons does this sign present for me? and *How do my feet embody this part of my nature?*

As you read from your chosen vantage point, keep an eye out for what it means to you. Which characteristics are feeling strong and robust? Which could be better developed? Be as honest with yourself as possible to get the greatest benefits from the book.

Everyone has strengths and susceptibilities, neither of which is good or bad. Overly strong has its fair share of problems (like muscle strain, bullish behavior), as does being overly susceptible (like shoulder dislocation, lack of confidence). You need a balance of both to be healthy. You need to stand strong *and* sway in the wind, like the proverbial reed that outlasted the oak tree in a storm because it was able to bend and not break. Jot down your strengths and susceptibilities as they become more apparent through what you read.

Need help choosing which characteristics to nurture? Which to bring into a better balance? When reading, note the descriptions of body regions and star sign characteristics that resonate with you the most—those that instantly stand out as big yeses or nos. A strong reaction either way indicates aspects that need greater consideration. Over time, your practice will change as you are called to embody different traits. They all live within you and, at different times in your life, will need to be expressed in different ways. So feel free to return to each chapter for reference throughout your life. Each reading will reveal something new.

Most importantly, this book is intended to take you on a journey through the cosmos as it lives both around and within you. Proceed, then, with a sense of exploration as befits an astronaut, along with an open imagination about how this wellness guide can best serve you. Our universe, galaxy, solar system, planet, and bodies are nothing if not magical, and accessing them is practical magic at its best.

Note

1. David C. Lindberg, *The Beginnings of Western Science: The European Scientific Tradition in Philosophical, Religious, and Institutional Context, Prehistory to A.D. 1450* (Chicago: University of Chicago Press, 2007), 2–3.

1

As Above, So Below

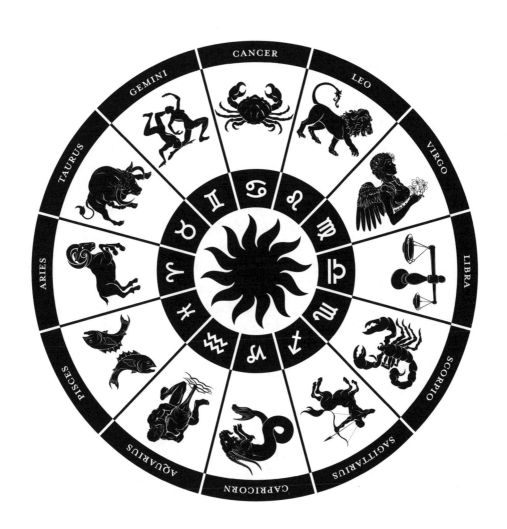

The *you* that you see in the mirror is a body borne of millions of years of anatomical evolution—a head, a torso, arms, legs, and more that define our species. But what about the rest of you? The parts of you that are not visible or tangible but that define you to your very core? (And by *core* we mean more than your abdomen!) These bits and pieces of your body are so much more than physical form: they are the living, breathing embodiment of your hopes and fears, strengths and susceptibilities, dreams and disappointments.

Civilizations throughout history have looked to the stars to empower our understanding of ourselves and our world. For aeons, our ancestors saw no distinction between earth and heaven, the natural and the divine; the stars were reflected within the regions of the body and, correspondingly, offered an insightful guide to life's inner workings. Let's look at our hands as an example: You likely see two functional appendages, while our ancient Greek predecessors looked at their hands and saw a gift from the gods—a gift from Zeus, ruler of the gods, to be exact. This gift was in the form of twin sons, known in Latin as *Gemini*, represented as a constellation of stars the sun passes through every year (May 21–June 20).

According to the ancient Greeks, your two hands represent the Gemini connection to realms both mortal and divine, and the communication between one and the other. When you consciously attune to your hands (using them enough but not too much, engaging them in proper alignment, and keeping them strong yet supple), you evoke the best of your own Gemini characteristics no matter when you were born, such as great adaptability and communication. And likewise, if you are not in balance, then Gemini's susceptibilities—such as feeling scattered—may predominate.

The study of this relationship (between heaven and earth, celestial bodies, and human affairs) became the study of astrology. It is a mathematical art and science that developed out of people's daily observations and experiences for thousands of years. And as illustrated by the Gemini myth above, our ancestors believed that the physical and nonphysical worlds were united, that ancient gods pervaded, animated, and informed the earthly world.

Without our modern, scientific knowledge, their surroundings—and the wisdom derived from them—were poetry. Storms were not the result of fluctuating meteorological conditions, but the outcome of mighty clashes between the gods. Earth did not arise through a happenstance combination of gases, but was born from the womb of a great Mother. Love was not an activation of dopamine-rich areas of the brain, but a shot from Cupid's bow. There was no distinction between matter and spirit, nature and divine. Gods regularly influenced, and were influenced by, earthly affairs—and there was no greater place to witness the workings of these divinities than the night sky.

As Above...

On a clear and dark night, a couple thousand stars may be visible to the naked eye. To the trained eye, these stars combine to form twelve constellations, each with its own story and sign.

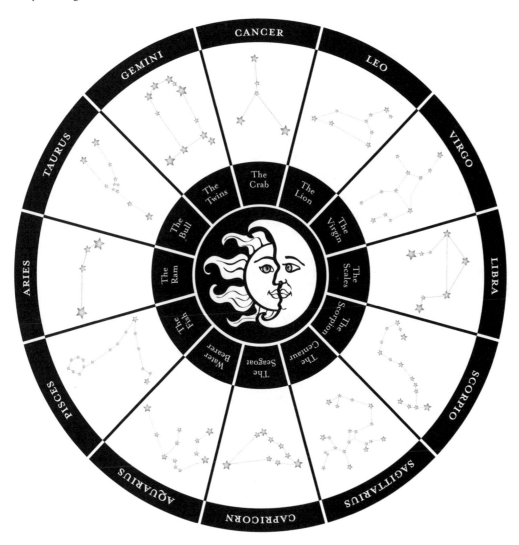

These twelve constellations lie along the sun's path, known as the ecliptic plane, forming a starry belt called the zodiac. In principle, the sun travels through one constellation a month, working its way through the entire zodiac in a year. (Since the sun is not actually moving, its apparent path is the trajectory it appears to make in the sky, based on the vantage point of an observer viewing the sun from Earth, which rotates as it orbits the sun.) Our current system for understanding the zodiac derives from ancient Greek geographer-astrologer-astronomer-mathematician Claudius Ptolemy who, around the second century BC, wrote the astronomical treatise describing over half of today's eighty-eight known constellations (the better our telescopes become, the more constellations we have been able to see). These days, the International Astronomical Union (IAU) updates astronomical understanding via a consortium of scientists that convenes to set standards for stars and space. Needless to say, given a fourteen-billion-year-old universe, there is still a lot left to know! For this book's basic astrology purposes, however, the primary players are the planets and signs.

> At the time of publication, the IAU designates eight planets: Mercury, Venus, Earth, Mars, Jupiter, Saturn, Uranus, and Neptune. Pluto now belongs to the relatively new and growing category of dwarf planet, along with Ceres, Eris, Makemake, and Haumea.

According to the IAU's updated requirements for planet status, eight planets currently exist. That said, astrology counts eleven, including Pluto (plus additional objects like the Sun and Moon—the luminaries—which are not planets, per se, but exert a similar effect).

> Whether or not Pluto is called a planet, it remains the same physical and metaphysical entity. Astronomically, it is a lump of ice and rock that is associated, astrologically, with a deep sense of power and evolution. Pluto's discovery in 1930 helped astrologers explain the rise of individual and societal events, like psychoanalysis and nuclear power... qualities that bear a striking similarity to its mythic namesake, the Roman god of the underworld.

Each planet represents a dimension of your character. For example, Mars represents action, a powerful force that helps drive you toward your goal whether during a marathon or an argument. Venus, in contrast, characterizes you as a lover and underscores the qualities that attract you to your partner from the get-go. All the planets are present throughout your birth chart.

If the planets function like actors on your living stage, think of the signs as roles that the planets play as they travel through the zodiac. There are twelve zodiac signs of 30 degrees each, equally dividing the 360-degree celestial sphere (see page 3). And while your sun sign might be the most prominent, all twelve signs live and express themselves within you.

Second to your sun sign, two other signs factor prominently into your disposition. The moon sign (the sign the moon was journeying through at your birth) reveals your inner self, needs, emotions, and fears; it is the part of you that those closest to you see. The rising sign (the sign on the eastern horizon when you were born) is how you project yourself into the world and often how the rest of the world sees you, including the impressions you leave on other people. This is why a fiery Sagittarius sun sign might appear like a caring Cancer to her spouse and a balanced Libra to her friends.

As a planet travels through each of the zodiac signs, it is influenced by each sign's distinct characteristics. For example: Gemini's role is communication. When the planet Mars is traveling in Gemini, he brings his trademark style of action into the realm of communication; he might therefore become a verbal powerhouse, aggressively advancing his cause in a way that would make any debate team proud. On the other hand, Venus traveling in Gemini is a charming orator, expressing her message with the grace and ease that befits a beauty pageant queen.

With its complexity, astrology becomes much more than pop culture prediction or predestination. The original intent behind astrology was to optimize the human condition by drawing the connection between the planets and the stars to life on Earth, to use the language of the sky to learn from the past and make the most of the present and future. Throughout time, astrologers have used astrological information for a variety of purposes, including informing important political decisions, forecasting weather patterns, fortuitously timing events, and caring for one's health. In other words, astrology has been used to answer *why*, *when*, and *how* versus *what*. And the same holds true today: each horoscope may function like a self-help guide, a way of understanding your true self and living it accordingly.

It is more accurate, then, to think of astrology as some combination of descriptive and prescriptive. It depicts who you are at your core and recommends the environment most conducive to living fully in that knowledge. It is like nature and nurture all in one. For years, science has known that nature affects nurture and is increasingly finding that nurture affects nature too. In fact, the fledgling field of epigenetics is devoted to understanding more of nurture's role. Thus far, scientists have ascertained that while your genes do not change, the signals that tell your body when to express those genes can be altered by environmental factors like food, relationships, and stress. In other words, what you choose to eat, the quality of your marriage, or the toxicity of your environment might affect whether your predisposition toward heart disease is expressed and how. Astrology, likewise, understands mankind is influenced by genetic and environmental factors but expands our understanding of environment to encompass the solar system as well.

Throughout history, different cultures have adopted different forms of astrology. For instance, Western astrology defines the signs based on the position of the spring equinox and emphasizes the sun sign within the natal chart. In contrast, Vedic astrology (of Hindu origin) uses fixed stars as its reference and may emphasize karma and the moon sign. Chinese astrology places emphasis on yearly—versus monthly—cycles, and on associations with elements (wood, fire, earth, metal, water) and animals (such as dragon, horse, monkey).

The greatest emphasis in Western astrology is placed on your sun sign, and this book maintains the same. So while the characteristics of all of the signs live within you, those of your sun sign (the sun's zodiac sign at the time of your birth) are the ones that predominate in your true nature. For instance, if you were born between July 23 and August 22, the sun was in the sign of Leo. Your natural disposition, therefore, includes Leo's strengths, like courage, ambition, and magnetism, and susceptibilities like pride and narcissism. Note that your sign's traits do not exist to the exclusion of others—a Leo can certainly be philosophical like a Sagittarius or analytical like a Virgo. You embody all the signs' traits, but those of your sun sign shine the brightest.

How does knowing this help you? Well, if you are an apple, you are always going to be an apple—never an orange—whether you want to be or not. And to be the best darn apple you can be means being aware of and living according to your true, apple nature. Similarly, if you are a Leo and you know that you are tailored to the spotlight, then choosing a career as a subway conductor is likely not conducive to your long-term success. Sure, you can do it—but it goes against the inherent light-loving and gregarious nature of your sign. For the happiest and healthiest life, learn to work *with* your true nature, developing your strengths, learning from your susceptibilities, and finding the appropriate balance between your sun sign and all other eleven signs within you. Astrology can offer this deeper insight and personal guidance.

...So Below

And the study of astrology does not stop there! In fact, astrology provides many ways to bring its teachings to life, from guidance (such as being aware of communication and transportation troubles during a Mercury retrograde) to grains (via foods and herbs associated with the qualities of each planet). But your body is the approach to astrology that is literally at your fingertips.

Your body is amazing. It is a miracle of Mother Nature some six million years in the making. Standing in front of a mirror, you can see its shape is a five-pointed star made up of one head, two arms, and two legs. Together, these structures form the *you* with which you are most familiar. Yet the true beauty of your body is not its individual parts but their greater, functional whole. Walking, running, skipping, jumping—together, your bones, muscles, and more orchestrate a symphony that allows you to operate as you see fit. However, we currently live in a society in which most of us know how to operate our laptops better than our legs—a world in which synchronizing takes place between our calendars and computers more frequently than between our head and neck. Forget about considering the body as an integrated whole—many individuals do not even know its parts exist. That is, until a body part stops behaving as it is supposed to and aches, breaks, or otherwise fails to perform.

But it wasn't always this way. Once upon a time, the whole is all that was seen. A focus on structural parts did not exist until anatomists like Galen of Pergamum wielded scalpels to systematically dissect bones, brains, and veins and detail them in enormous bodies of work that influence science today. But back then, when Galen delineated the body's parts, he also correlated them to a person's spirit (as previously identified by Plato). The heart, therefore, was viewed as both the source of the body's circulation and the seat of a person's passion; the brain begot the body's nerves as well as the soul's mind. For Galen, proof of divinity was in the physical pudding.

And so it is with astrology. Each of the twelve zodiac signs governs a region of the body—starting with Aries at your head and ending with Pisces at your feet, with all the other signs in between. You might be familiar with the Middle Age illustration of the Zodiac Man, depicting the twelve zodiac signs superimposed on the human form.

What this figure refers to is the body as man's key to the cosmos, the idea that each sign's energy lives within and can be accessed through the related body region. In this way, all of the character traits, strengths, and susceptibilities of each zodiac sign do not have to remain just concepts. They can all be brought to life so that

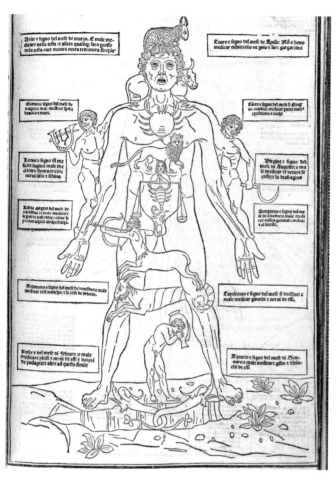

*Johannes de Ketham, "Zodiac Man," Fasiculo de medicina
(Venice: Gregori, 1943)*

who you are is aligned with what you do. Bringing your own, personal Zodiac Man to life is like walking the talk in regard to well-being.

Your body can literally bring to life the story of the stars. It is not as hard to access as you might think, because the stars already live and breathe within you. Really. Man is made of the same substance as stars, which is the literal truth. Stars consist primarily of helium and hydrogen, and during their life-death cycles over the past billions of years, they have fabricated almost every other element as well, including carbon, nitrogen, and oxygen. Lo and behold, these essential elements are the same ones that comprise life as we know it, the same ones found in the soil, grass, food . . . and you. Hydrogen, for instance, is part of the water molecule (H_2O) that constitutes over half of your body's mass. Carbon is distributed throughout the double strands of your DNA. Nitrogen forms a vital part of your body's proteins. And oxygen is the

There are many depictions of the Zodiac Man, but the original illustrator is still unknown. Most of the drawings date to the Middle Ages, although the first text referencing the concept is older, appearing in Marcus Manilius's works of 15–20 BCE. His works, in turn, were based on wisdom passed down from his predecessors. How did they ascertain the relationship between body and stars? Well, for the majority of known human history, the natural and the divine were simply two sides of the same coin. Our predecessors' conventions of thought were different than ours, and we cannot look back to a different age and ascribe our modern mentality to them. Their proof was primarily based on life experience, not empirical research (like how you subjectively know that sleep is good for you without having to be told by a scientific study). So they knew it by virtue of living it.

primary fuel for trillions of your cells. In short, you live because stars died and recycled their material as you.

This might be your first encounter with the idea that you embody both the matter and the spirit of the stars, but it is an age-old relationship that predates even Babylonian records. Look at the following chart to see how the zodiac signs correlate to your body parts.

You can check out the most prominent signs in your chart, like the sun, moon, or rising sign, but remember that all twelve zodiac signs live within you! That is, in fact, what the hermetic axiom "As above, so below" means—the heavens are reflected here on Earth and the Earth, in turn, reflects the heavens. Which means if you have a body region, then you have the story of the corresponding sign alive in you. For instance, your loving Leo heart and cautious Capricorn knees.

There is no helium in the human body but, along with hydrogen, it makes up about 98 percent of the known matter in the universe.

Sign	Body	Sign	Body
Aries	Head	Libra	Lower back
Taurus	Neck	Scorpio	Sacrum
Gemini	Arms, forearms, hands	Sagittarius	Hips, thighs
Cancer	Chest	Capricorn	Knees
Leo	Upper back, heart	Aquarius	Ankles
Virgo	Abdomen	Pisces	Feet

Whether or not you realize it, all of the zodiac signs' characteristics present facets of you—facets that are yours to express if you so choose. The question, then, is which facets to express and how. How will you bring the story of the stars to life through your bodily form?

2

Head of the Ram

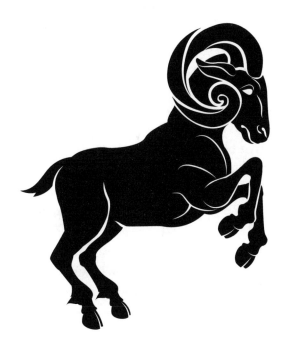

♈ ARIES

Birth date: March 21–April 19
Body region: Head
Theme: Assert Yourself with
Active Awareness

T he zodiac is a cycle that starts with Aries and ends at Pisces, only to begin again. As the first sign of the cycle, Aries highlights the individual. It represents your metaphysical birth into the world by introducing *you*, who you are and what you are here to do. It is your sense of self. A recognition that you possess your own unique head and feet, wants and needs. While you are a product of your environment, you are also distinct from it, and Aries immerses you in individuation by helping you tune in to your truest self and consciously assert it in your surroundings.

Your Body: Head

Headstrong is a term that applies well to Aries, not least of all because the head is the sign's related body region. Indeed, the Aries head *is* strong. Actually, everyone's head is strong in order to protect the contents therein, a.k.a. your brain, which is the command center of your body. The bony structure of the head is composed of the skull, which is a collection of twenty-two bones. Touch the top of your head, though, and it feels like only one bone because they are fused together at suture joints that allow your cranium to feel and operate like a solid whole.

It is not just the baby's head that needs to be supple for birth but also the mother's pelvis. Typically, to accommodate the way humans walk on two feet, the pelvis needs to be stable and narrow; during delivery, however, hormones like relaxin help the ligaments loosen so that the pelvis may widen.

Why so many bones, then, if all you really need is one strong one? Because several floating bones are more flexible than one solid one. This flexibility allows a baby's relatively large head to fit through a relatively small birth canal; and once the baby has entered the world, the flexibility also allows room for his brain to grow. If you feel the top of a baby's head, you can feel the floating bones in an area called the anterior fontanelle, a membranous opening between the frontal and parietal bones that may not fuse for almost two years.

There you have it: the very first part of you to enter into this world is your head, and it is literally and figuratively wide open. The Aries in each of us must therefore maintain a clear head to be aware of all that we might experience so we can pick and choose our own adventures. Otherwise, we can be trapped in a life not of our own making, which presents a problem for Aries energy, since it exists to forge its own path.

Fortunately, the head sits atop one of the most mobile regions of the body—the neck. Your neck moves the head through almost 180 degrees of side-to-side rotation, which allows its sense organs to appreciate a great deal of your surroundings. Indeed, your eyes, ears, nose, mouth, and skin all reside on your head, and it is their

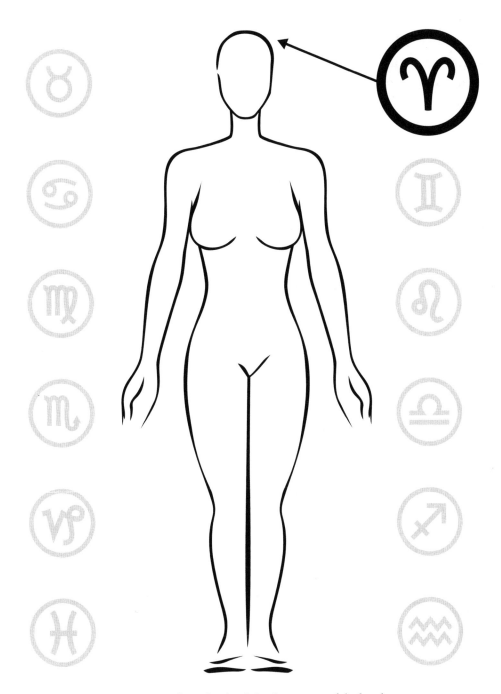

See appendix C for the skeletal structure of the head.

incoming impressions—along with the brain's processing of them—that ultimately inform your reality. They provide the external information that your mind uses to mold your internal one, and vice versa. For instance, without having ever seen or heard of a gym, you would not know it exists. Once you are aware it exists, however, you can incorporate it into your regular health routine. It is key, then, for our Aries nature to attune to as much of our environment as possible so we can choose the elements that work best for us.

How much of your environment do you receive? Try this to find out:

1. Stand up and stroll around your surroundings for one minute. Interact with them as you ordinarily would. Do not read further until you return.
2. After you return, write down ten things that you saw.
3. Take stock of how you interacted with your surroundings: What did you see? Did you incorporate the ceiling, floor, and walls in your purview, or did you restrict your experience to what was in front of you?
4. Now stroll around again, trying to see more actively and fully.
5. After you return, write down five new things that you saw. What elements did you notice that you did not before? What did that require of you?

Many individuals keep their heads fixed in one direction while they walk around. With eyes gazing ahead (or at a phone), they are oblivious to everything their surroundings have to offer. Looking only at the ground, or listening only to their internal dialogue, they miss the grass, the people, the sky. Senses set in one direction receive only one set of information. And yet, from the evolutionary perspective, your senses exist for a reason—to receive lots of data from your environment so you can decide how to respond, if at all. In other words: if you do not realize that a lion is behind you, chances are you will be eaten. So your head, along with its sensory organs, and the brain it contains, facilitates your awareness.

The Stars: Aries

Assert Yourself with Active Awareness

Have you ever heard the saying "How you do one thing is how you do everything"? If you have not, take a moment to consider it: How do you walk down the street—

purposefully or aimlessly? When you talk to friends, do you end your sentences with conviction or a rising intonation? How you walk, talk, and otherwise choose to carry yourself through your day are all examples of how you assert your presence on this Earth.

Make no bones about it, the Aries is here to assert—definitively and decisively. He is here to declare his presence to the world with a purposeful "I am!" and a will to survive that is reflected in the very season of his birth—spring. Like the seed in spring that knows it will eventually grow to be a tree, every Ram is a pioneer, pushing onward and upward with purpose. Aries energy is always directed forward with strength of will. Envision this sun sign's namesake, the Ram. With its two large horns, the animal is not easily deterred. And neither is the Aries spirit. This spirit is a formidable commitment to true self and purpose—shoulds and expectations be damned. And it is from this commitment that true power shines. Not power as defined by society at large, but the powerful fuel of a fire that resides deep inside you, a force that is here to assert exactly who you are and what you are here to do.

We live in a society of mores and norms, opinions and expectations that exist at both conscious and subconscious levels, and they affect us all to varying extents. For instance, when your mind told you to attend a certain college in order to have a certain career in order to make a certain amount of money in order to succeed . . . how much of that plan was actually yours? It is a difficult question to answer because the individual-collective interplay is woven throughout our lives and our decisions therein. But it is possible to be more or less affected and, in this regard, the Aries falls on the side of less, on the side of exerting himself on society, and potentially scornful of society's influence altogether.

This self-absorbed focus is needed for the zodiac sign charged with defining autonomy or, more succinctly, the *I*—it is needed for the sign associated with our thoughts, our minds, our heads. But do not confuse an emphasis of the *I* with arrogance. Can the two be connected? Absolutely. But they do not have to be. The *I* can also live in its most simple state—a recognition that the self is an individual, distinct from others in the crowd. Which means that, as you survey your surroundings and hear what others have to say, you do not lose sight of who you are and what you want. Take, for example, the Aries civil rights leader Booker T. Washington. Washington was born into slavery and, after emancipation, worked his way through school during an era when everyone told him it was neither his place nor possible. But he was so dedicated to becoming the best that he could be that he not only made it through school, but he ultimately became the first leader of the Tuskegee Institute as well as an advisor to United States presidents Theodore Roosevelt and William Howard Taft—making Washington one of the first black political leaders in the country. His self-actualization approach mirrored his beliefs as he advocated for progress through education and industry—not by protests against segregation laws, as was the norm at the time. His approach was controversial, but Washington stuck to his guns and, as a result, was able to build rural schools and business leagues for African Americans, none of which had previously existed.

In this way, Washington is a model Aries and a model for anyone wanting to embody Aries's strengths—to focus on their *I* and what they want. He knew his needs and pursued them despite the odds. The Aries developmental psychologist Abraham Maslow says, "What a man *can* be, he *must* be. He must be true to his own nature. This need we may call self-actualization. . . . This tendency might be phrased as the desire to become more and more what one idiosyncratically is, to become everything that one is capable of becoming."[1]

In other words, we are all here to self-actualize, to define *and* assert our own paths. And it does not matter what path, as long as it is our own. It is the Aries nature we embody when we speak our minds. A nature that cannot and must not be constrained by others' perspectives, even if we risk disapproval from parents and peers in the process. Should we listen to others' perspectives? Of course. But we must use those perspectives as information, as data points that represent different aspects of what the world can offer. With so many aspects, the more we are aware of them, the better. Recall that Aries, as the start of the zodiac cycle, is its metaphysical newborn. And just like a newborn, our Aries nature attends to the aspects of our surroundings that call our names and direct the attention of our awareness, albeit with the bonus of rational thought layered on top of instinctual reaction.

Abraham Maslow proposed his hierarchy of needs in a 1943 paper. Today, the hierarchy is famously pictured as a pyramid of basic needs including (from bottom to top): physiological, safety, belongingness and love, esteem and self-actualization. A later and controversial addition includes self-transcendence.

How much of your environment are you aware of? Awareness is conscious perception of the world around you, from the seen (such as a physical store) to the unseen (an emotion like anger). It is a state of perception that exists in both passive and active forms. Passive awareness refers to the reception of sensory experiences without trying to, wanting to, or even realizing that you are. For instance, with peripheral vision you see one hundred degrees laterally, sixty degrees medially, sixty degrees upward, and seventy-five degrees downward outside of your central vision; this means that even if you are walking along the street staring at your phone, stores will enter your purview even if you are not looking directly at them. Active awareness, on the other hand, is an intentional tuning in; it is you walking down the street paying attention to each store that you pass. This willful engagement is important to cultivate because the more paths an Aries is aware of, the better able he is to choose the one that works for him. The one that best affirms his own thoughts and interests.

That said, while Aries energy is most attuned to what his surroundings can do for him, he needs to keep one eye open to his impact on them as well. Otherwise, he may get lost within the machinations of his own mind, his own wants and needs, oblivious to those of others. This is one peril of being driven exclusively by the Aries nature—as we try to be more independent, we run the risk of being too much in our own heads.

The best cautionary tale about an Aries whose at-all-costs individuation leads to all-around destruction is called the Quest of the Golden Fleece, the Greek myth associated with the Aries constellation. Jason, a confident and courageous young man, auspiciously emerges from the woods to assert himself as the rightful king of a previously stolen throne. Long story short, he is given the opportunity to regain his royalty in return for a ram's fleece. This special fleece is thought to be unattainable, but Jason—like any good Aries—leaps at the challenge. He assembles a fleet of heroes on a ship called *The Argo* and recovers the fleece.

His success, however, is not without struggle, which he overcomes with the good graces of Medea. Medea is a sorceress who, with a shot from Cupid's bow, falls in love with Jason. She makes great sacrifices to help him (like killing her own brother) and ultimately leaves the rest of her family to become Jason's wife. Jason promises Medea that she will be worshipped for her deeds when they return to Greece.

However, when the hero returns home, he is blinded by royal ambitions. He abruptly disavows Medea, minimizes her role in his success, and chooses to wed another woman in order to add renown to his throne. Medea, upset, uses sorcery to take everything from Jason, including the life of his new bride. Ultimately, Jason ends up angry, alone . . . and totally unable to see how his own thoughts and actions led to his demise. Sigh. If only he could have seen his situation for what it was—versus what he wanted it to be—he would have achieved the full glory of his birthright.

If you see only what you want to see, you will ram through life with blinders on. Blinders can be a healthy tool to reduce distractions and enhance focus, but they only work if you first have a chance to glean what lies above, behind, and below. Garnering a full spectrum of information helps ensure that the chosen road is the right one for you and includes an acknowledgment of the surrounding world.

Lessons

Your mind creates stories from the input your head receives. For instance, if you read about a new diet plan and it makes intellectual sense, you might decide that it is a good option for you; your food story subsequently becomes "I eat only XYZ." If this story is aligned with your personal truth, then you will be eating according to what your mind wants and your body needs. If your story is unaligned, however, you will be spending your days shopping for, thinking about, and eating foods that serve your intellect better than your physical form.

Whether they focus on food or Foucault, your mental machinations may arise from a variety of sources—self, family, society, school—and the Aries is here to decipher their personal relevance and authenticity. It is self-centeredness at its best, as long as the Aries's self arises from your highest truth and acknowledges that yours is one of many. If you are able to achieve this precious balance, you are effectively living the zodiacal lesson of Aries: to define and assert your independence in synergy with your surroundings.

If, however, you are unable to identify yourself and how you fit with those around you, the Aries shadow side will emerge. Your inner Ram will become irritable; things will never seem to go as planned and he will blame others for this perceived failure. Refusing to question his internal convictions, he will not understand his lack of external achievement. He will see something wrong with his surroundings versus the outdated stories in his head and the need for greater awareness. When this occurs, the Ram's energy will feel thwarted. He will feel as if, lacking external execution, his formidable thoughts and plans are forced to remain inside his head. In nature, rams butt heads with their enemies; in this case, it will be the Aries Ram who is butting heads not only with others but with himself too. As the body region related to Aries, the head retains its energy. Energy that is unable to be constructively released will remain stuck inside, manifesting as frustrated thoughts and feelings. Tension will build and, as more energy becomes stymied, the Aries's head will feel increasingly stuffed.

Physical manifestations of stuffed Aries energy may include:

★ Headaches
★ Migraines
★ Head cold
★ Ear infections
★ Teeth grinding, infections

★ Irritated sinuses
★ Facial blemishes
★ Stuffed nose or head
★ Tight jaw muscles

If, on the other hand, you know exactly who you are and what you are here to accomplish, your Ram will be a formidable force. Without maintaining an appropriate amount of humility, however, the Ram might explode with assertion and plow over anyone or anything he perceives as standing in his way. He might lash out willy-nilly at those who dare question him . . . ultimately causing more self-harm than good. And instead of listening to counsel from others, he will continue to stubbornly adhere to only his own advice. Failure is not typically an option for our Aries side but, in this scenario, it becomes a self-fulfilling prophecy.

Physical manifestations of an explosive Aries nature may include:

★ Headache
★ Migraines
★ Runny nose
★ Tooth pain, infections

★ Diminished hearing
★ Eye infections
★ Facial blemishes
★ Hair loss

How aware is your head? Whether it feels stuffed, explosive, or somewhere in between, the key is listening to your body and giving it what it needs. Awaken your inner Aries with the questions and exercises that follow.

Your Body and the Stars

The following will serve as your personal guide to embodying the Aries stars. Use them to assert yourself with active awareness.

Questions

★ Who are you, really? Write down a list of adjectives that describe you at your core (for example, intelligent, passionate).

★ Look at your list and circle the top three that you want to assert more during your day. What action would you need to take to make that happen? What prevents you from asserting yourself that way in the first place?

★ When you assert yourself, what effect does it have on others in your surroundings (like friends, environment)? Can you assert yourself more effectively?

★ Are you actively aware of your surroundings? When you walk down the street, do you keep your head fixed in one position or do you intentionally look around?

★ How do your surroundings help or hinder you on your path?

Exercises

Head Nod: For Stronger Self-Assertion

Know who you are and make it happen! Start with the Pilates head nod, which helps strengthen the musculature around the head so that it sits properly atop your neck. A well-set head speaks volumes about your sense of self. It is stable and well supported, not rolling around like a wobbling Weeble. This stability confers a firm conviction (a good head on your shoulders, if you will) that helps you fight for who you are and what you are here to do.

1. Lie on your back with your knees bent and feet flat on the floor. Elongate your arms by your sides, palms facing down.
2. Find a neutral position with your head, so that it is level with the ceiling. In this position you should retain the natural curve of your neck.
3. On an inhale, tilt your chin down toward your chest. Feel this movement as an elongation in your neck versus a compression.
4. Exhale, returning your head to neutral position.
5. On the next inhale, tilt your chin up and back. Again, move with a feeling of elongation in the neck.
6. Exhale, returning your head to neutral position.
7. Repeat ten times, ending with your head in neutral position.

The movements of your head should be slow and small, so that in both flexion (chin titled down) and extension (chin tilted up), your neck feels supported. In moving your head, make sure not to neglect the neutral position; this position approximates how you should position your head when standing.

Standing Forward Fold: To Renew Your Sense of Self and Surroundings

Every day you walk around with an upright perspective—the natural state of affairs as an upright human being. Sometimes, though, your worldview needs to be turned upside down! You need to see the same things in a new way in order to grow. Bring a new perspective to what your senses receive with this standing fold.

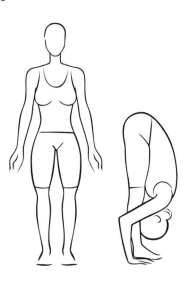

1. Stand in a neutral position with feet hip distance apart and arms elongated by your sides. Tune in to how you feel.
2. On an exhale, slowly roll your upper body down into a folded position, starting with your head, followed by your neck and then upper back, middle back, and finally, lower back. Roll down one vertebra at a time until your hands reach the floor. If they do not reach the floor, place your hands on the front of your legs for support.
3. Relax into your maximum fold, wherever it is. Make sure there is no tension in your head or neck. You may close your eyes.
4. Nod your head yes several times. Shake your head no. Nod your head yes again.
5. Remain in the fold for a few more seconds, allowing the blood to flow toward your head.
6. If your eyes are closed, open them to look around your environment from your new perspective. Pause for a moment to take it in.
7. On an inhale, slowly roll up to a standing position by reversing the direction of the way you came, one vertebra at a time, through the lower back, middle back, upper back, neck, head.
8. When you have returned to your standing position, close your eyes and pause. Sense any differences in how you feel now compared to the beginning of the exercise. For instance, do you feel tingling? More open? Relaxed?

Sound Meditation: For Active Awareness of Your Surroundings

Move beyond your mind's machinations into expanded awareness. A greater awareness of yourself and your surroundings is always within you; sometimes you just need to quiet the mind to find it. Meditation quiets the mind through disciplined focus. Researchers speculate that primitive hunter-gatherer societies may have discovered a meditative focus while staring at the flames of their fires. Through subsequent centuries and societies, meditation evolved into a more structured practice. For instance, some of the earliest Hindu scriptures, called Vedas, mentioned meditation techniques about five thousand years ago, and the Buddha made meditation a central tenet of his philosophy around 500 BCE. There are many ways to meditate and even more points of focus. The following meditation actively focuses your attention on the sounds from your immediate environment. In this way, the mind moves away from its stories and toward your greater surroundings.

1. Choose a space and time that is free from interruption. Turn off your phone ringer and set an alarm to alert you when this ten-minute meditation is over.
2. Find a comfortable seat on the floor, sitting cross-legged upon a cushion, pillow, or block if needed (if cross-legged is not possible, find an easeful position sitting upright on the floor; if this position is not possible, sit on a chair). The best seat is one that can healthily support you for the next ten minutes.
3. Rest your hands in your lap, palms facing up. Gently close your eyes.
4. Focus your mind on one sound occurring around you like traffic, crickets, or a running faucet. Keep your attention on the sound by simply listening to it.
5. When your mind wanders, catch it as soon as possible and bring it back to the act of attuning to your environment and concentrating on a sound. Do not feel defeated if your mind wanders—most do. Focusing takes regular practice, which is why meditation is considered a practice.
6. After your alarm sounds, stay seated with your eyes closed and pause for a moment. Reflect on the experience before you continue your day.

If a ten-minute meditation seems daunting to you, feel free to practice this meditation in any time interval that seems doable (for example, two or five minutes). The most important part of any meditation is simply showing up to do it. The length of your meditation will naturally increase over time.

Neti Pot: To Clear Your Head

The neti pot has been used by yogis for *jala neti*, or nasal cleansing, for thousands of years. You might be more familiar with its modern equivalent, nasal irrigation. Whether then or now, the practices are similar and involve streaming a saline solution through the passages of your nose. While a simple practice, it requires a certain temerity to try it. The benefits, however, are well worth the effort and are believed to include reduced allergy and sinus symptoms, clearing of nasal debris, and improved smell and taste. See for yourself how this ancient practice helps keep your entire head clear. How—even if your head does not feel stuffed—there is always the opportunity to make it more open and sense things you did not before.

1. In a neti pot, mix no more than a ¼ teaspoon of salt with lukewarm water. Use the purest salt available to minimize irritation (like unrefined sea salt).
2. Lean forward over the sink and turn your head to one side.
3. Gently insert the spout of the pot in the upper nostril so it forms a comfortable seal.
4. Breathe through your open mouth.
5. Slowly lift the pot so the water flows in through your upper nostril, out of the lower nostril, and into the sink. Use half the pot.
6. When you have used half of the pot, blow gently and repeatedly into the sink to clear the nasal passages. Do not pinch your nostrils.
7. Repeat on the other side using the remaining half of the solution.
8. After blowing into the sink, dry your nose with a tissue or towel.

Note: Beginners should expect to experiment with this technique a few times before finding the best position. While you are experimenting, water might drip down your throat, a similar sensation to getting water up your nose. To minimize chances of this occurring, do not talk or laugh while using the pot. Though you will probably experience some discomfort from it being a new and unfamiliar sensation, if it is truly uncomfortable for you, discontinue use.

Exfoliating Mask: To Show Your True Self

Your skin cells regenerate approximately every twenty-seven days, which means that every month, you are literally presenting a new face to the world. The value of this self-renewal has been understood throughout the ages and practiced in the form of facial masks. For instance, Cleopatra was purported to have used Dead Sea mud as a clay mask, and royalty in Chinese dynasties were reported to have ground gemstones, like pearl and jade, into tonics for the face. If you do not have access to ground gemstones, do not despair. Simple ingredients like oatmeal and honey work well too. This oatmeal mask will gently exfoliate your skin, encouraging its inherent renewal. Use it to reflect a renewed sense of self or when you wish to invoke one.

1. Buy steel-cut oatmeal.
2. Cook one serving of oatmeal as directed on the package.
3. Let oatmeal cool to a lukewarm temperature.
4. Clean and dry your face as usual. Apply oatmeal as a layer to the entire face and leave on for ten to fifteen minutes.
5. Rinse off mask with cool water and a washcloth.

Bonus: You can add honey (about 2 tablespoons) between steps 2 and 3 for greater moisturizing.

"I Am" Exercise: For Confidence in Who You Are

The Aries motto is "I am." And, sometimes, you have to say it to believe it. Use the three adjectives that describe you at your core (culled from the top two questions on page 20) or pick three others that you wish to invoke, to remind yourself who you

 A phrase similar to "I am" was coined by the Aries mathematician-philosopher René Descartes: "I think, therefore I am." Given his zodiac sign, it is fitting that this mental powerhouse used thinking to validate existence; surely, there are many alternatives, such as "I feel, therefore I am," "I breathe, therefore I am," and so on.

really are. For instance: "I am powerful," "I am handsome," "I am intelligent." Whichever words you choose, say them to yourself—out loud—while looking in the mirror. Repeat as many times as you need to believe it. Then go into the world and be it!

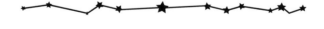

Summary

Your head is the region related to Aries. Featuring five senses (and the brain that processes them), it governs your perception of the world along with your place in it.

★ Aries is the first sign of the zodiac cycle. Its energy pertains to who you are and what you are here to do . . . along with the will to make it happen.

★ If your assertive Aries nature gets stifled or, on the other side of the spectrum, is unchecked (by you!), your head might experience different symptoms (e.g., stuffiness, runny nose, headaches).

★ Align your inner Aries through questions, exercises, and activities that focus on your head. Use them for self-renewal, which comes part and parcel with the Ram and his birth season, spring.

Note
1. Abraham H. Maslow, *Motivation and Personality*, 2nd ed. (New York: Harper & Row, 1970), 46.

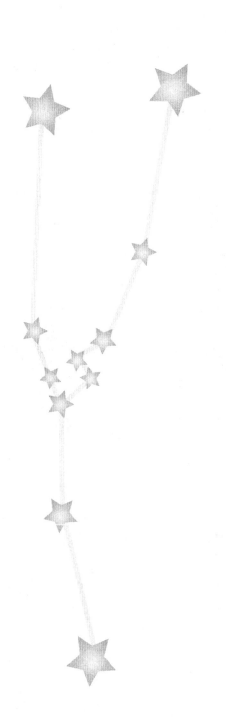

3

Neck of the Bull

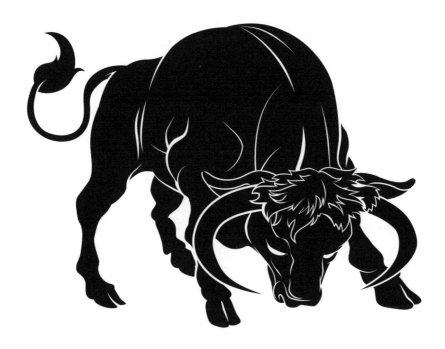

♉ TAURUS

Birth date: April 20–May 20
Body region: Neck
Theme: Transcend the Material by
Exalting the Sensual

aurus, as the second sign, builds on what Aries knows. She has grown a bit from her newborn Aries days and is now a toddler. Able to identify her *self*, she can project that sense onto the world and does so by grabbing, touching, and tasting everything in sight. Aries comes into the world with the motto "I am," and Taurus follows with "I have"—she sees what the earth has to offer and wants to make it hers. Indeed, as an earth sign, Taurus inherently loves the material realm and all its treasures—like lots of money, timeless art, good food, and great sex. Earth is a playground for the senses, and appreciation of the sensory experience at the most exalted levels is what the Taurus is here to express.

Your Body: Neck

The bull is a distinctive-looking bovine, notable for a large frame (weighing an average of two thousand pounds) that includes a large neck. The bull's neck is such a prominent region that in medical jargon, *bull neck* is its own term—referring to an individual whose neck is enlarged (typically due to hypertrophied muscles or swollen lymph nodes). Given the association between the bull and its neck, it may not be surprising that the neck is the body region related to the zodiac's Bull, Taurus.

The neck is a narrow structure located between the head and back, composed of seven vertebral bones (cervical vertebrae). These bones are just one part of a vertebral column that spans throughout your back and neck and is commonly referred to as your spine. The spine has different types of vertebrae, and the ones in your neck are the most delicate. Each cervical vertebra has a thin structure to facilitate range of motion punctuated by holes to permit the passage of vessels and nerves to and from the head. But while delicate, the neck is not weak: your neck supports your bowling ball–sized head while simultaneously moving it. In fact, the cervical region has the greatest range of motion of the entire spine, up to ninety degrees of rotation in each direction. This range of motion moves your head and allows it—along with its eyes, ears, nose, and mouth—to sufficiently sense your surrounding environment.

Helping your head receive sensory input, however, is only half the battle. The neck is also responsible for communicating what you make of the input to the rest of the world. It does this via the vocal cords, two membranous folds of tissue found in

> ♉ The necks of almost all mammals—including humans, bulls, and even giraffes—have seven vertebral bones.

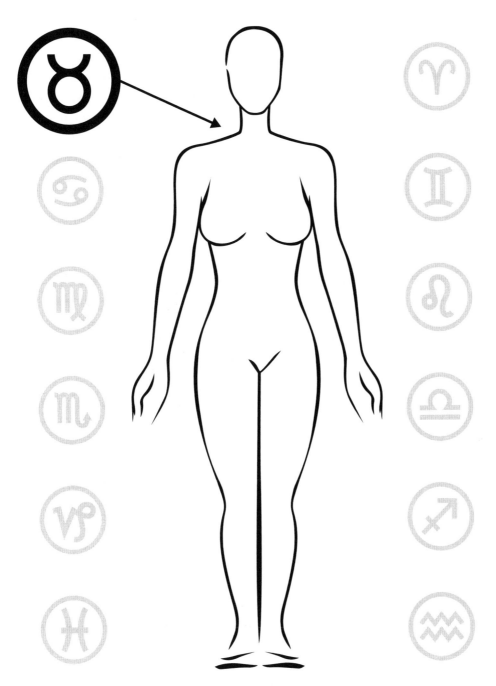

See appendix C for the skeletal structure of the neck.

the trachea that are evolution's gift to gab. Mechanically, the folds are used to form air's vibration into sound and sound into word.

Words are one of your primary modes of expression. Words communicate internal thoughts, feelings, and sentiments to the external world. The words you choose, along with how you choose to say them, not only reflect how you see yourself but also shape your idea of it. It is imperative, therefore, that the words Taurus says express the full extent of her nature, from the practical to the passionate, from the corporeal to the cultured. Not one side of the spectrum, but both. The Bull needs to dutifully inquire into interest rates on loans as well as exalt in the beautiful decor of her home. If your inner Bull expresses only part of your sentiments, you will be expressing only part of yourself. And the rest of your thoughts and emotions will not magically disappear; rather, they will remain within the neck, lodged in the form of stress or strain.

Neck strain, unfortunately, occurs all too easily, and can be caused by a variety of reasons. Physically the joints, muscles, and ligaments of your neck incur stress as a result of the improper positioning of your head and neck—like when you sit, stand, walk, or read with your head inadvertently jutting forward or cocked to one side. Because optimal vocal expression entails proper positioning of the vocal cords (which occurs when the neck is properly positioned between the head and trunk), if you disturb the alignment of your neck (and the cords therein), you similarly disrupt your ability to express. Take a moment to ascertain the state of your neck. See for yourself how well it is aligned between your head and trunk:

1. Stand in front of a mirror and turn sideways for a profile reflection. Stand as you normally would if you were not paying attention to your posture (no cheating!).
2. Rotating your head as little as possible, look toward the mirror and observe if your head and neck project forward.
3. If they do, bring them back into alignment over your trunk so that your head, neck, and back rest in one straight line, with your earlobes positioned over the top your shoulders. If your shoulders are curved forward, straighten them as well.
4. Notice the difference in this new alignment, compared to the prior one. This alignment is closer to your ideal.

Many folks in modern society stand with a fixed forward flexion of the head. In this position the head and neck protrude in front of the trunk, as if leading the show. You may be in this position when walking down the street or sitting in front of your computer screen. But the head, while an important player, is not meant to perpetually protrude. It is meant to sit directly atop the heart, with the neck bridging the two. That way, the neck expresses the best of both worlds—the sentiments of the heart and the senses of the head.

The Stars: Taurus

Transcend the Material by Exalting the Sensual

To *transcend* is to surpass some form of limitation. In mathematics, for example, transcendental numbers like Π or e surpass algebraic limits; in transcendental meditation, the practitioner enters states of awareness that surpass those of daily consciousness; in transcendental philosophy (whose founding father, Immanuel Kant, has Taurus as both sun and rising signs), knowledge is transcendental if it goes beyond an object to your mode of knowing the object. No matter which way you slice it, transcendentalism allows the mind to perceive your physical reality and then says, "Hey, there's still so much more." This mentality is especially poignant for our Taurus nature. Taurus relishes the material world, but her enjoyment of it is called to extend beyond the matter at hand.

The Taurus in each of us delights in material things that she can have and hold, and she works hard for them. Like her related constellation, the Bull, every Taurus possesses a persevering and practical nature. No wonder, then, that the Taurus loves all the good things money can buy. They represent rewards for her endurance, for sticking through a job to make sure it is well done. But fully realized Taurus energy will transcend the material reality and appreciate its higher nature, extending beyond the physical form and into the realm of emotions, mind, and spirit.

Take, for instance, food. Food, like the rest of the material world, is made of matter and is something that can be consumed simply for its own sake. Or it can provide a transcendental experience, no better exemplified than with *la madeleine*, the small cake that the author Marcel Proust (a Taurus moon sign) made famous in his classic work *Remembrance of Things Past*. Upon having a madeleine with his tea one day, Proust describes his experience with the cake as not just the intake of batter and butter but as something that transported him through time and space. One delicious bite brings back the taste of his childhood breakfast on Sundays, the sound of a church's steeples, and fond feelings for his deceased aunt. In other words, the madeleine provided Proust with a feast for his senses. A realm of experience that went well beyond the ordinary capability of carbohydrates.

Of course, sometimes, to paraphrase Taurus psychoanalyst Sigmund Freud, a madeleine is just a madeleine. Objects can certainly be enjoyed in their own right, without having to evoke something more. Indeed, daily life would be very challenging if every bite of lunch brought you into a heightened state of awareness. But this is the state our inner Taurus is called to embody. Because her disposition is so intimately tied to the earth, the Bull must learn not to get stuck in her earthly nature. Instead, she is here to use the physical form as a foundation for the even greater experiences that exist beyond what the hands can hold and eyes can see.

 Atoms are almost entirely empty space. And yet, if you took all of the atoms in our world and removed the space between them, a single teaspoon of the resulting mass would weigh about five billion tons.

From the book in your hands to your hands that are holding it—the material world both constitutes and surrounds you. The building block of this material world is the atom, billions upon billions of which create the world that you can see, taste, touch, hear, and smell. And while atoms are not solid entities, the interaction of their electromagnetic forces presents the illusion of solidity, so that you perceive a world full of things.

Taurus is at home in the realm of things, especially luxurious things. From fine jewelry to leather gloves, and from gourmet food to exotic fragrances, she loves possessing luxury. She derives great comfort from their enduring quality and seemingly solid nature. It is as if having lots of things helps her remain connected to the biggest thing—the Earth.

Buddha has long been associated with Taurus. In fact, he is believed to have been born, enlightened, and deceased during the months of the sign (April and May). If this is true, then by creating a philosophy centered around nonattachment, he learned—and taught—the highest of Taurus's lessons.

Being connected to the earth brings good things. But *caveat emptor*! Our Bull nature may become attached to our belongings. We may forget that the fun in having is not actually about the object itself but the experience or learning it brings. We are greater than any one—or even the sum—of our possessions. Possessions may help facilitate experiences that make us happy, but that happiness ultimately arises from within.

So don't become your own King Midas, the mythological king who turned everything around him into gold (including his own daughter!) and was subsequently unable to enjoy any of it. You should absolutely enjoy the hard-earned fruits of your labor. But if obtaining them is your end goal, you will never feel satisfied no matter how much you have. For instance, you will work hard to buy a fancy car, stay at the same job to afford its maintenance, stay longer in order to buy a second one, and ten years later realize that you have never driven the cars on outdoor excursions or joy rides. You will be so focused on acquiring the physical things that you will miss the greater pleasures they bring.

The physical level offers many greater pleasures. As discussed in the Aries chapter, your senses bring data through your sense organs (eyes, ears, tongue, skin, nose) to your brain for processing. For instance, when you read a poem, light rays reflect off its words and travel through your eye's cornea, iris, and lens to meet the retina, where nerve cells (rods and cones) convert the light into electrical impulses. The optic nerve then sends these impulses to the brain where an image is produced, thereby allowing you to read. This complex chain of events is remarkable in itself. But if you have ever read a poem—or any written word—you know that your experience with what you are reading is even more robust. Because in addition to physically seeing the words, you have likely thought or felt something. Perhaps you formed an opinion based on an essay, enjoyed a book, or were inspired to further study by an article you read. An infinite array of impressions accompany the words that your eyes see.

In this way, poems are more than words written on paper, just as pictures are more than images. The greater beauty of poems and pictures—as well as anything classified as art—lies in the stories they express and the sentiments they inspire. Which means that there is more to your senses than just a physiologic reaction, as your physical senses elicit mental, emotional, and spiritual sensations as well. In this capacity, your senses exist in an exalted form—beyond what the eye can see, nose can smell, ear can hear, etc. An exalted sense is therefore heralded both on the material plane and higher, as in the realms of thought, feeling, and inspiration.

Seeing, smelling, tasting, touching . . . while the Taurus in us is great at experiencing her senses at their basic level, she is here to evoke their exalted forms. She does not necessarily need to write poems or paint pictures herself, but she benefits from being surrounded by Earth's beauty—all of its magnificent colors, textures and sounds. Sensual sensitivity provides the perfect complement to her

In astrology, the term *exaltation* refers to a planet's relationship with a zodiac sign in which its energies and potential are amplified. For instance, the moon's exaltation sign is Taurus, so when the moon is exalted as it moves through Taurus, its qualities relating to the five senses are heightened.

enduring, hardworking, materially oriented nature. It is the side of her that gets to stop and smell the roses after spending months tending the garden. And in modern society—let alone for the nose-to-ground Bull in each of us—stopping to smell anything is no easy feat. It takes intention and practice. But even the actual bovine lifts its neck up from the earth to gaze upon the heavens; so it is for the Taurus to elevate our desires for the physical into an exaltation of the sensual.

Lessons

Relishing the gifts your senses receive does not require millions of dollars or the life of a retiree. It is about finding delight through the material versus being weighed down by the mundane. And while the mundane matters, there is more to life than just that. Every object your senses behold possesses a value that exceeds its physical existence. It possesses an experience, a thought, an emotion, a lesson, or some greater sensation for you to derive from it. In this way, everything is both matter and spirit, allowing you to find a little bit of heaven in each object here on Earth.

This heightened sensuality is like a sixth sense—a sense of greater beauty that is inherent to the Taurus nature in us all. Do not be fooled by how you commonly consider the bull, as bovines are not typically viewed as refined. The Taurus Bull is so much more than nose-to-the-ground. This sign is one of the most tender, romantic, and sensual of the zodiac. While renowned for her persistent and enduring efforts, the Bull's greatest gifts lie in her ability to look up and enjoy what is around.

It is crucial, therefore, for the Bull in you to embrace her tendency toward a higher ideal and to express who she is in all of her material-minded *and* sensual-seeking glory. She needs to discuss the tangible merits of an object while also delighting in its greater appeal. She should propound on the practical and also promote play. If this part of your nature fails to appreciate the breadth of experience each sense has to give, your self-expression will feel constricted as part of your Bull is held at bay. The part that is here to roam in delight will be nowhere to be found or artificially held down by fear of losing her ground. Sure, the Bull is a naturally grounded animal, but even this bovine can be overly so.

Physical manifestations of a fixed Taurus energy may include:

★ Neck tension
★ Stiffness or aching

★ Restricted range of motion
★ Crackling or crunching sensations with movement
★ Others: Cough, sore throat infection, thyroid imbalance, unsteady voice

The deep roots of the Bull are essential to her need for security—which is a deep-rooted need. However, if she mistakes security for the pleasures that sensuality brings, she will find herself on a perpetual wild goose chase. Possession after possession will accrue as your Bull tries to cobble together stability. Whether owning lots of shoes or purchasing watch after watch, your Bull might rely on a continuous influx of physical goods in order to connect to her sense of ground. But without the proper ground, underlying anxiety and fear—related to lack of security—will ultimately win out.

Physical manifestations of a desirous Taurus energy may include:

★ Weak neck muscles
★ Hypermobility
★ Instability
★ Constant popping or urge to crack neck
★ Others: Thyroid imbalance, raw throat, unsteady voice

How expressive is your neck? Whether it feels fixed, desirous, or somewhere in between, the key is listening to your body and giving it what it needs. To stretch a tight neck or strengthen a weak one, awaken your inner Taurus with the questions and exercises that follow.

Your Body and the Stars

The following questions and exercises will serve as your personal guide to embodying the Taurus stars. Use them to transcend the material by exalting the sensual.

Questions

★ What percentage of your day do you spend obtaining objects (for example, working or shopping)? What percentage of your day do you spend enjoying them?
★ Is there one sense you rely on more than others? Are there any senses you neglect? How could you engage more of your senses throughout the day?

★ How easily do you find a greater beauty in your daily affairs? What is your daily version of stopping to smell the roses?

★ When do you feel the most free to express yourself? Who are you with? Where are you located?

★ What people, places, and things hinder your freedom of expression? Try to notice if, when your expression feels hindered, you are more inclined to touch your neck.

★ When you speak, what do your words typically express? Some form of planning, preparation, or recalling? Or appreciating, enjoying, and feeling?

Exercises

Isometric Neck Strengthening: For a Strong Physical Foundation

Take care of your physical needs. Cultivate strong roots so the rest of you can securely grow. Even the tallest sunflower has its foundation deep in the ground. The following isometric exercise strengthens the neck through its full range of motion to bring greater support to the basic senses of your head and your ability to express them.

1. Start in a relaxed standing position.
2. Place the palms of both hands evenly on your forehead. Keeping your chin parallel to the ground, press your forehead forward into your hands and hold for a slow count of ten.

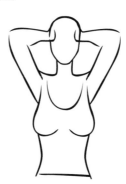

3. Place your hands on the back of your head and push your head into your hands, keeping your chin parallel to the ground. Hold for the same count of ten.

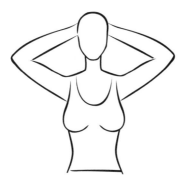

4. Place your right hand on the right side of your head, above your right ear. Push your head into your hand, as if bringing your ear to your shoulder. Hold for ten counts. Repeat on the left side.

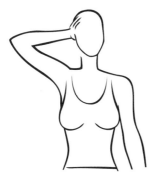 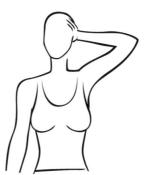

5. Place your hand on the right side of your head, around the area of your temple. Keeping your chin parallel to the ground, rotate your head to the right, pushing your temple into your hand and your hand into your temple. Hold for ten counts. Repeat on the left side.

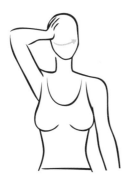 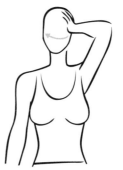

6. Relax your hands by your sides and *gently* shake out your head and neck.

This series strengthens your neck through the resistance of your hands. You therefore have the ability to exert as much, or as little, resistance as you like. The more you counter the movement of your head with pressure from your hands, the smaller your head and neck movements will be. No matter what level of resistance you create, be sure to keep your shoulders relaxed and away from your ears.

Head and Neck Circles: To Open into Greater Sensation

There is a whole lot of world out there, and a supple neck will help you sense it and appreciate what you sense. Move your neck through its full range of motion so that your head sees, tastes, touches, smells, and hears more than before. And be prepared to communicate about everything that you ingest! An open neck is also more readily able to express.

1. Stand with your feet hip distance apart, with a slight bend in your knees. Arms are hanging by your sides. Head is in its neutral position, with chin parallel to the floor.
2. Keeping your neck and shoulders relaxed, nod your head toward your chin and then roll your head *slowly* to the right, making sure you move through all the directions—front, side, back, side, front. Perform the circles as if you had a ball the size of a fist between your head and neck (this will prevent you from moving your head through an excessive range of motion). Repeat five times, ending with your head in its neutral position.
3. Reverse directions, rolling the head toward the left. Repeat five times, ending with your head in its neutral position.

Once you feel comfortable performing the circles, close your eyes to move deeper into the exercise. For an added bonus, add breath: every time your head rolls toward the back, take a slow, deep inhale; when your head rolls forward, enjoy a slow, deep exhale.

Mantra: For Fuller Expression

Learn to express your voice in new ways using mantras. Chanting mantras is an age-old technique that uses primal sounds to convey sacred meanings. For instance, the mantra *HAM* invokes the qualities of the energy center connected to the neck (*vishuddha chakra*). By repeating the sound, you tune in to the energy and lessons of your neck. Mantra, while renowned for its Hindu roots, is also found throughout Buddhism, Sikhism, and Jainism. And the concept of hymns and chants is found in even larger circles, including Judeo-Christian culture, in expressions like "In the beginning there was the Word" and "Amen." In ancient Egypt, the Taurus was even called "the interpreter of the divine voice." Use the following mantra practice to express your own.

1. Choose a space and time that is free from interruption. Turn off your phone ringer and set an alarm to alert you when this two-minute meditation is over.
2. Find a comfortable seat on the floor, sitting cross-legged upon a cushion, pillow, or block if needed (if cross-legged is not possible, find an easeful position sitting upright on a floor; if this position is not possible, sit on a chair). The best seat is one that can support you for the next two minutes.
3. Rest your hands in your lap, palms facing up. Gently close your eyes.
4. Feeling the vibration originate in your chest, produce the sound *HAM* (pronouncing the *a*, as in *father*). Allow the sound to be long and expansive as it rises from your chest and up through your throat. Feel the *mmm*'s vibration as it leaves your lips, as with the word *humming*. Repeat the mantra, allowing one pronunciation to flow after the other.
5. After your alarm sounds, stay seated with eyes closed and pause for a moment before getting up. Feel the residual vibration throughout your body.

For greatest effect, practice the mantra every day for at least forty days. As you gain a sense of the sound and its rhythm, your meditation may progress so that you chant it more softly. Ultimately, once you are familiar with the sound and its vibration, you may chant it silently to yourself.

Nature Walk: To Transcend the Material

The Bull is born to appreciate Earth's bounty. Enjoy your earthly nature with a walk in the wild—whatever park, hill, or brook inspires you most. As you walk, engage all of your senses as you attune to your environment: smell the air, hear the birds, see the sun's rays, and feel their warmth on your skin. Now go one step further and apply the Taurus's sixth sense of greater beauty. For instance, apart from warmth, what other sensations does the sun invoke? Childhood memories? Happiness?

Relaxation? Notice what sensations arise for you on the walk that were not present before you started. This ability to tune in to your senses can be yours with practice. After a few focused nature walks, you will find yourself increasingly privy not only to your basic senses but also to the greater places they lead.

Bonus: Use your neck to express by whistling or humming a song while you walk. The Taurus singer Ella Fitzgerald once said, "I don't want to say the wrong thing, which I always do . . . I think I do better when I sing."[1]

Adorn Your Neck: For Enhanced Expression

The décolletage is the upper part of a woman's torso, comprising her neck, shoulders, upper back, and chest. And even though it is simply one part of her body, what it says—by how it is adorned—is so much more. Whether with the exposed cleavage of the Baroque era or the high necks of the Victorian, what a woman does with her décolletage may serve as a statement of both fashion aesthetics and social norms. And the same is true for men. Wearing a tie may be appropriate in one venue or inappropriate in another, and in either case say more about the wearer than he might suspect. Consider what your décolletage says about you:

★ How is your neckline currently adorned (turtleneck, necklace, bow tie, V-neck sweater, scarf)?
★ What is its adornment (or lack of) expressing? How could you adorn, expose, or hide your neckline to more accurately express you?
★ What sensations arise when you wear a low-cut shirt, loosen your tie, or drape a silk scarf? Even without having to put them on, what connotations do they invoke?

For one week, pay special attention to how you dress your neck every day. Play around with it and see how wearing—or not wearing—something different subtly changes your type and level of expression. No doubt, the peanut gallery will have their own opinions. Note them, but ultimately decide for yourself how your neckline is most suitably expressed.

Stop and Smell the Roses: To Exalt the Sensual

It takes practice to appreciate the finer things in life, and there is no better time to start than now. Here is one way to do it:

1. Buy yourself a bouquet of roses "just because."
2. Put the flowers in a vase on top of a table that you pass regularly.
3. As you pass them, pause and delight in their symphony of sensations—their rich color, the velvety feel of their petals, and their fragrant scent.
4. Focus on their scent by closing your eyes. Lean toward a rosebud and inhale deeply, breathing in its fragrance. Feel where it takes you.
5. Repeat one more time.
6. Nothing lasts forever and one day your roses will be gone. Appreciate them while you have them.
7. Extend your enjoyment of your roses after they wilt by adorning your home with dried rose petals (on your bedspread, as part of a well-set dinner table, or in a bubble bath).

This practice is not to be undertaken by anyone with flower allergies.

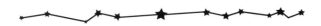

Summary

★ Your neck is the region related to Taurus. With the vocal cords located within, it expresses how you see yourself and, simultaneously, shapes your idea of it.
★ Taurus is the second sign of the zodiac cycle. Its energy pertains to living and celebrating the full extent of who you are, from the material to the sensual.
★ If your aesthetic Taurus nature becomes overly concerned with security or desirous of sensual pleasure, your neck might experience different symptoms (e.g., tension, weakness, cough).
★ Align your inner Taurus through questions, exercises, and activities that focus on your neck. Use them to help your inner Bull grab life by the horns . . . and enjoy it!

Note
1. Jim Moret, "Ella Fitzgerald Dies at Age 78," CNN Web Archive, June 15, 1996, http://web.archive.org/web/20061129231320/http://www.cnn.com/SHOWBIZ/9606/15/fitzgerald.obit/index.html.

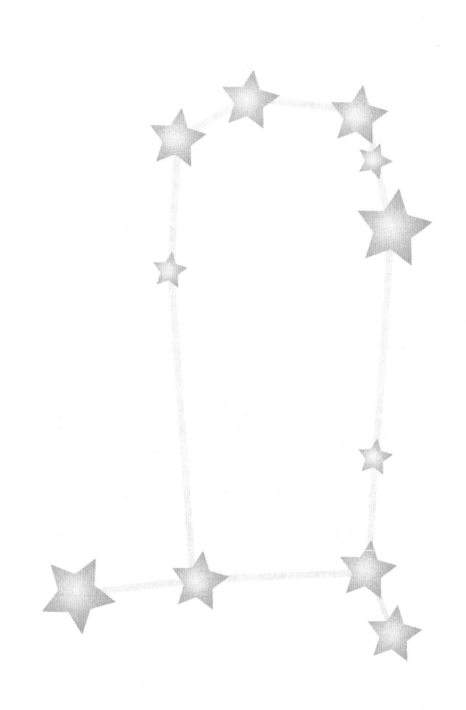

4

Hands of the Twins

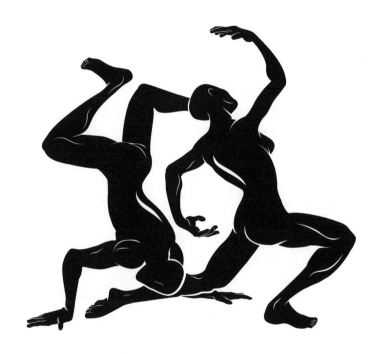

♊ GEMINI

Birth date: May 21–June 20
Body region: Arms, Forearms, and Hands
Theme: Serve as Messenger of
Your Illumined Mind

A ries and Taurus, the first two signs of the zodiac, delineate you as an individual, as a drop of water separate from the rest of the sea. This personal foundation is important because, come Gemini, your now-solid *me* begins to recognize that it belongs to a greater *we*. It recognizes that you actually reside within a larger body of water—while separate, you simultaneously belong to a greater whole. Gemini is therefore the first sign of the zodiac to not operate as self versus other but to start bridging the two. Blessed with a brilliant mind and the dexterity with which to share it, Gemini is here to deliver his individual ideas to the greater world.

Your Body: Arms, Forearms, and Hands

In the title of the chapter, "Hands of the Twins," *hand* is actually "shorthand" (pun intended) for the entire upper extremity; you have two upper extremities, or limbs, and each is composed of an arm, forearm, and hand. Gemini is the only zodiac sign that is related to more than one musculoskeletal body region.

♊ Aries's and Taurus's more self-centered focus is represented by a singularity found throughout their signs—defining *one* self, represented by *one* constellation (like Ram or Bull), with *one* related body region (like head or neck). Gemini, in contrast, gives birth to the concept of *two*. It introduces *two* individuals (the other in addition to the self), is represented by a constellation of *two* beings and a body region consisting of *two* upper extremities (inclusive of *two* arms, forearms, and hands).

Yet these different regions work together to accomplish a unified goal—to allow the hands to connect to objects in space. Your arms and forearms, while useful in their own right, exist so that you can wave hello, shake hands, open doors, strike matches, and perform a whole host of gestures that allow humankind to communicate with its surroundings as only humankind can.

Let us start with the arms, the region of the upper limb that connects to the rest of your body, as well as connecting you to your greater environs. Once upon a time, our primate predecessors used this ability to connect to vast areas of their jungle as they swung from vine to vine. Currently, your arms allow you to connect in other ways—grabbing groceries from a shelf above you or picking flowers. Their extensive reach comes from the shoulders, two ball-and-socket joints that are the most mobile joints in the body (with the humerus forming the ball and the scapula the socket).

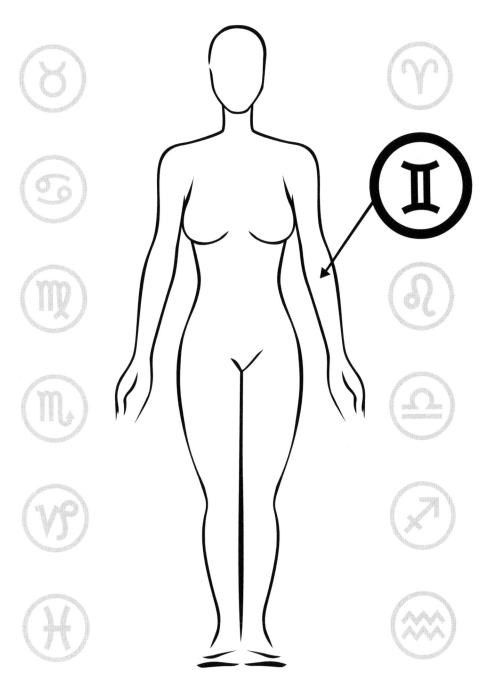

See appendix C for the skeletal structure of the arm, forearm, and hand.

From each arm arises the forearm, a region that does not typically receive much attention but gets its job done. The forearm extends between the elbow and wrist joints. Its two bones, the radius and ulna, allow movement at both joints (albeit much less than at the shoulder), but their equally important role is to take the force from the arm and transfer it to the hand. This transition—along with its mitigation of force—helps control and refine the movements of your hands.

In contrast to the gross movements of the arms, the movements of your hands are fine—think about how your hands can ever so slightly change their grip to enable you to hold a pencil, insert a key into a lock, or sew a button. This dexterity is enabled by the approximately thirty bones, eleven sets of intrinsic muscles, and four regions of joints found in each hand. This intricate structure is distinctive to our species and features a thumb that—because it is not bound by ligaments to the other fingers and attaches to the hand at a different angle—is opposable.

> ♊ The word *thumb* is derived from the Latin *pollex*. Therefore, muscles that move the thumb tend to have *pollicis* in their names, like the thumb flexor muscle, *flexor pollicis longus*. Pollex is not to be confused with Pollux, the giant star with an orange hue in the constellation Gemini, and the mythological brother of Castor.

All in all, the hands serve as the body's ultimate messengers thanks to their infinite array of movements and manipulations. Heck, hands are so handy at communication that millions of individuals use them to speak entire languages through signing.

It bears repeating, though, that the hands—while the stars of the Gemini show—do not work alone. They work together with the arms and forearms to connect your internal ideas to the external world. For example, if you have a great idea for a new internet company, one of your first steps is to write it down . . . after your arms, forearms, and hands enable you to obtain the paper and pen in the first place. Gripping the pen, your five fingers bring intangible thoughts to tangible reality as they scribble a business plan. With plan in hand, you are ready to present your idea to an investor.

> ♊ It's no surprise that the Latin root for hand, *manus*, is also the root of the word *manifest* . . . which is exactly what your hands do when they take a thought (like an idea for a company) and make it evident to the eye (like writing a business plan).

Imagine the presentation in its perfect form—as your lips champion your idea, you are likely using your arms, forearms, and hands to passionately gesture, to give greater life to the cause. Now, imagine giving the same presentation with your arms firmly folded across your chest. Even though you are saying the same words, your body is broadcasting an entirely different message, all because of some flexion and extension at your shoulder, elbow, and wrist joints.

In this example, your upper limbs served to develop your idea and deliver it to the world in two different ways, which brings us back to the Gemini's role as messenger. What is your message? How are you delivering it? How are you using (or not) your arms, forearms, and hands to communicate its concepts to the people who need them? Many people proceed through the day unaware of their extremities' utility; as a result, arms flail and fingers are closed in doors. How connected are you to the movements of your upper extremities? See for yourself with this simple exercise:

1. Choose a position, either seated or standing. Fold your arms across your chest.
2. Which arm did you fold first, right or left? Did you need a moment to think about the answer, or did you instinctively know?
3. Repeat the gesture in slow motion and notice which arm folds first.
4. Relax your arms by your sides.
5. Now, fold your arms across your chest using the other arm first.

Chances are that you are better connected to the arm that you folded first, and it is your dominant one (which, statistically speaking, is your right side); folding your nondominant arm first might have required a momentary pause before you began. This occurs because your two limbs are asymmetrical. You have developed one side more than the other because you eat, write, and brush your teeth using predominantly one hand. But this does not mean you cannot cultivate the riches of the other. It is the Gemini juggling act—with a dual nature (and handedness), how do you access both sides of your nature so you can benefit from A *and* B, not just one or the other? And if you have the facility for both, what do you gain by relying on one to the exclusion of the other?

> It is known that the right hand is ruled by the left side of the brain and vice versa. The reality of handedness, however, is far more complex, and it appears that a whole confluence of factors—neurologic, genetic, behavioral, physiological, societal—are involved, with further research warranted before any conclusions may be definitively stated. ♊

The Stars: Gemini

Serve as Messenger of Your Illumined Mind

There are many ways to be of service, to put yourself to a use that is greater than just your own. This utility can occur through many different means (such as helping a friend move, driving a bus, becoming a politician) and on many different scales (e.g., one-on-one, group, global). "Service" is action that exceeds personal utility or promotion. An action that extends from self to other.

Gemini brings the concept of service into the zodiac by introducing the "other." The other represents all those people in the world who are distinct from you, with their own thoughts, feelings, hopes, and dreams. Typically around age two a child recognizes that he is not the only one in the sandbox. Ultimately, he learns that he can better serve himself—and others—not by screaming but by communicating his desire to share a toy with words, like *want* or *no*. At the adult level, the learning is the same: you can either speak to hear your own voice or share your thoughts in a way that acknowledges those with whom you are conversing—typically a much more effective way to be heard, whether by friends at a cocktail party or clients at a marketing meeting.

Indeed, Gemini is here to serve others through communication. The Gemini energy is here to create and connect communities through ideas. But it bears repeating that the most important contribution to service involves the introduction of the other. Gemini is not the public broadcasting station of the zodiac, nor is his energy here to proselytize on behalf of a greater good—these endeavors relate to lessons learned farther along the zodiac wheel. The Gemini is simply here to share what is in his head with the world around him, even if his reasons are self-serving. That's okay. Everyone is allowed to benefit, not just to benefit the other—and our inner Gemini is here to remind us of this dual reality.

At this stage of the game, it is no longer you versus them, but you *and* them, a coupling that consists of a complementary pair. So while some individuals may view the world as black or white, heaven or earth, masculine or feminine, good or bad, higher or lower, etc., the Gemini sees both sides of any equation. This duality forms the foundation of his nature and, as part of the zodiac, exists within yours, too. Invoking your inner Gemini will help you live in a world that is good and bad, heaven and earth, simultaneously.

The beauty of recognizing duality is that you do not have to choose between self or other, but you can embrace them both. You can cultivate and enjoy your own gifts and also share them in a way that benefits others. For example, Walt Whitman was a Gemini poet whose poems, like those from his famous collection *Leaves of Grass*, transformed the field of poetry by introducing free verse. The field might have found itself stymied in rhythm and rhyme if Whitman had confined his poetry to a personal hobby and concentrated instead on his career as a typesetter for a local newspaper.

Of course, you do not have to be a Whitman in order to successfully serve. You might serve a stranger by engaging in cheerful banter on the subway, serve your family by telling fantastic stories at bedtime, or serve colleagues by penning an inspiring memo. Service is service regardless of audience size. And it works especially well for our Gemini nature when it involves communication.

A messenger communicates a thought or idea via a medium. Whether the medium is telegraph, letter, word, or fist, messengers have delivered news of every ilk since the beginning of time. Angels are some of our world's oldest messengers and, in fact, the word angel comes from the classical Greek word *angelos*, meaning "messenger." Even if you do not believe in angels, chances are you know that lore says their role is to deliver the message of the heavens to humankind—not a far cry from the Gemini Twins.

> One of Walt Whitman's contemporary poets and devoted students, Allen Ginsberg, was also a Gemini. Like Whitman, he was a nonconformist and used his keen intellect to introduce new ideology through the literary medium, ultimately becoming an icon of the Beat Generation and the subsequent counterculture movement it inspired.

The Gemini zodiac sign is represented by twins who are not angels but are earthly as well as divine. It is through this dual nature that they are able to serve effectively as messengers between the two realms. Indeed, they are here to bring the highest ideals of the heavens to life here on Earth. They are here to inspire humankind to be and do better with new thoughts and fresh perspectives. The origin of their role is well illustrated by a Greek myth, which, like the Gemini's versatile nature, has many versions. The most typical version begins with the birth of the Gemini Twins to one mother, Leda, from two different fathers. Castor, the twin born to a Spartan king, was mortal. Pollux, born to the Greek god Zeus, was immortal.

The twins loved each other and enjoyed many adventures together, including the Aries quest for the Golden Fleece (see chapter 2: "Head of the Ram"). On one of their adventures to a foreign land, however, Castor is killed. Some myths report his death is due to a dispute over cattle, while others say it is over women. Either way, Pollux is inconsolable and prays to die. Zeus grants his wish but with the condition that Pollux will live half his time beneath the earth (in Hades) and the other half in heaven. In one version of the myth, the twins are together all the time in both heaven and earth. In another, they are never together, as one occupies heaven while the other occupies earth, and then they change places. Whichever way the story is told, the Gemini Twins dance between heaven and earth, mortal and divine. When in heaven they relay the stories of earth, and while on earth they convey the spirit of the heavens.

And so the Gemini is everywhere at once. The Gemini nature is adaptable and can help us flit around any environment to both garner information and give it. Gemini energy is aided in all endeavors by ruling planet Mercury, which is associated with the Roman god of communication. Augmented with the planet's quick-witted energy, Gemini immediately sees and synthesizes situations.

He is also blessed with the gift of gab to communicate his perspective compellingly. Mind you, his perspective may sound flighty to his audience as he says one thing today and then something else tomorrow. But it is only because for any given situation he sees all aspects together—not a paradox, as it might outwardly seem, but the Twins' multi-faceted reality. And this nature in each of us can help us do the same.

> ♊ The planet Mercury was named for the Roman god who darted from place to place, and it is the origin of the word *mercurial*, which refers to volatile, flighty, or erratic behavior.

Good communication takes into consideration others' perspectives; inevitably, your words will affect those you are speaking to and you should intentionally invest in their effect. In other words, a good communicator is aware of not only what is being communicated but also how it is being received. Where is your message coming from? How are you delivering it? To whom are you delivering it? And for what end? With the natural ability to connect ideas, people, and ideas to people, it is of the utmost importance that we engage our Gemini so he fulfills this role in our lives with integrity. To be conveyed with integrity, a message needs alignment between its medium, audience, and origin. For instance, if the message is "love thy neighbor," chances are it will find greatest effect delivered by a priest on a pulpit, to a church congregation, as a teaching of Jesus Christ. On the other hand, the same message, printed on a billboard alongside of Interstate 95 as part of a real estate marketing campaign will likely be perceived as insincere and its intended effect lost.

An effective message has the power to change the world. Take, for instance, the unforgettable phrase of Gemini President John F. Kennedy's 1961 Inaugural Address: "Ask not what your country can do for you, ask what you can do for your country."[1] With seventeen simple words, Kennedy called his nation to action. His message was one of hope as he asked his countrymen to rise to the challenges ahead. He invoked courage and community and peace, concepts that are eternal, and indeed, the power of the message outlived the messenger.

An effective message—especially of the eternal variety—is typically one that was composed by an illumined mind. What, you may ask, is an illumined mind? You are familiar with your plain ol' mind, famous for its ability to think, rationalize, compartmentalize, and otherwise make sense of your world. It is the part of you that is reading this book and forming opinions on it. It is the part of you that perceives. Now imagine that your mind is capable of even greater ways of obtaining information. This higher mode of operation is the realm of the illumined mind. It is the part of you that just knows without having to figure it out, the part of you that can make sense of your reality in a way that is more vast, expansive, integrative—and mysterious—than the machinations of your regular, lower mind. It is the part of you that is connected to . . . who knows, really? but a source of wisdom seemingly greater than just yourself. It is the part of you that, without your having to think about it, will allow the information in this chapter to click, so that in a few days or weeks what you are currently reading will make sense in a new light.

You need both the higher, illumined mind and the lower, regular mind because they work together. Ideally, the higher-order connections of your illumined mind filter through your regular mind so that what you know comes from the grandest place possible, and you are then able to communicate that information in a way that is understandable to others. These days, however, this higher-lower mind partnership is more the exception than the norm. As many of us in the Westernized world spend hours in office cubicles, we tend to rely on the lower mind for the origin of our thoughts, questions, and answers as well as their execution. This is one reason that so many people are so tired by the end of the day—they are only using half of their mental resources! So it is high time to rebalance the equation by cultivating the higher mind.

Fortunately, the Gemini Twins are up for the task. The illumined mind is, after all, the Gemini superpower. This is the source of Gemini creativity and inspiration, the locus from whence your messages must spring. This is how Gemini helps us serve a greater good—by connecting to a greater part of your self and communicating it. To do this, though, you must invoke your inner Gemini to recognize your dual nature. Just as Gemini energy is calm and anxious, strong and weak, busy and lazy, it is also of the higher mind and the lower—and you must consciously choose to cultivate the higher.

Easier said than done, of course, but it is possible with practice. The practice of receiving a flash of inspiration and trusting it; having a bright, bold idea and sharing it even if it is new or outside of the norm. At first, working with two minds might feel like juggling—unsure of what is coming or going, with several balls at any given time between air and land. But at the end of the day, juggling is a game. Fortunately, your inner Gemini is blessed with this natural sleight of hand!

Lessons

A juggler uses both of his hands to keep his balls in the air. He probably was not born ambidextrous but cultivated the ability to use both sides evenly over time. Such is the lesson we learn from our Gemini: to recognize our dual nature and bring all aspects into balance. And the aspects we typically need to balance are the higher ones, most saliently our higher minds and our connection to the other, both of which are there waiting to be developed. Our other aspects—like connection to self and facility with the lower mind—are likely facile already.

If our Gemini is unable to fulfill this mission, then he might feel limited in who he is and what he is able to do, as if he has great ideas to give to the world and yet they do not seem to work once they leave his mind. For instance, if your Gemini nature relies too greatly on the lower mind as the source for ideas, then the ideas might fail because they are not truly what you are here to communicate, or they may not resonate with the higher ideals of the community. Or your ideas may be accepted and even be financially fruitful but leave your Gemini unfulfilled because they cater too staunchly to the status quo instead of putting something new out there. You might then feel grounded, weighed down, constricted—which goes against the very nature of this brilliant air sign.

Physical manifestations of a limited Gemini nature may include:

★ Shoulder tension
★ Shoulder, elbow, forearm, wrist, or hand pain
★ Upper extremity joint crackling or crunching sensation
★ Tight shoulder blades (scapulae)
★ Restricted or stiff shoulder, elbow, wrist, or hand movement
★ Poor dexterity

Your Gemini side will likewise feel unfulfilled if impaired in his ability to connect with people, if he ignores the other half of his equation. For instance, if your ideas are wonderfully imaginative but employed only for self-interest or self-gain. In this scenario, you might end up alienating others and feeling scattered without any solid, interpersonal connections. Or your ideas may simply lack practical application. This scenario occurs when the Gemini gets wrapped in the sheer brilliance or aptitude of ideas without questioning if they actually serve a broader audience. There is no doubt that many ideas—no matter where they originate from—are excellent. But if they do not fulfill a greater purpose, they will nonetheless leave your Gemini side feeling unsatisfied.

Physical manifestations of a scattered Gemini nature may include:

★ Hypermobile joints, especially shoulder, elbow, or finger
★ Weakness or instability of upper extremities
★ Protruding or "winged" shoulder blade
★ Excessive knuckle popping
★ Poor dexterity
★ Weak grip or handshake

How well do your upper limbs communicate and connect? Whether they feel limited, scattered, or somewhere in between, the key is listening to your body and giving it what it needs. To stretch tight upper limbs or strengthen weak ones, awaken your inner Gemini with the questions and exercises that follow.

Your Body and the Stars

The following will serve as your personal guide to embodying the Gemini stars. Use them to serve as a messenger of your illumined mind.

Questions

★ What high-level message(s) are you here to share? For whom are they intended (individuals, communities)?
★ How do you share your message (through poems, pottery, PowerPoint)? How would you like to share it?
★ When you communicate, do you talk with your hands? When you shake hands with others, what message do you send (confidence, passivity)?

★ In what ways do you use your arms, forearms, and hands to bring your ideas to life?

★ What was your most recent inspiration or idea? How frequently do you share your ideas? How frequently do you act on them?

Exercises

Hand & Wrist Figure Eights: To Deliver Messages with Ease and Fluidity

This exercise is a modification of basic hand and wrist circles. The fluid movement involved in creating a figure eight with your hand provides a simple stretch that moves the wrist through a range of motion it does not necessarily experience every day . . . but should. These movements are quick and easy, and they can be done in a variety of locations, even an office setting as a brief computer break.

1. Sit on a chair with both feet on the floor, back straight, chin level with the ground.
2. Flex your right elbow to ninety degrees and make a figure eight shape with your right hand. Allow your fingers to lead the movement as they draw the shape in space.
3. Make ten slow figure eights. Then reverse directions.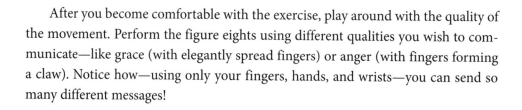
4. Repeat on the left side, both directions.
5. Shake out both hands.

After you become comfortable with the exercise, play around with the quality of the movement. Perform the figure eights using different qualities you wish to communicate—like grace (with elegantly spread fingers) or anger (with fingers forming a claw). Notice how—using only your fingers, hands, and wrists—you can send so many different messages!

Plank Push-Up: To Connect and Communicate with Strength

This powerful position is a great strengthener for your entire upper extremity, especially the muscles surrounding the shoulder joint. Strong arms will help you connect your ideas to your surroundings with conviction (which you especially need when proposing ideas from the illumined mind!). If you are not able to perform this exercise in proper alignment, use the modification below to decrease the amount of weight your shoulders, elbows, and wrists bear.

1. Start in a tabletop position on your hands and knees. Your wrists should fall directly under your shoulders, forming a straight line between wrists, elbows, and shoulders; the fingers of each hand should be firmly planted and spread out. Your torso, head, and neck should be parallel to the floor with eyes gazing down and slightly ahead.

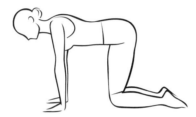

2. Center your weight between your upper and lower extremities. Engage your core, curl your toes under, and extend your legs. You are now in the plank position. Hold for at least one round of breath.

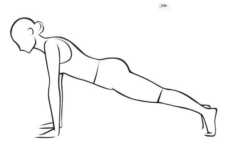

3. On an exhale, flex your elbows to a maximum of ninety degrees. Only bend so far as you are able to maintain the integrity of the plank position (no caving of the upper or lower back allowed!). Hold for at least one round of breath.

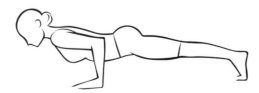

4. On an exhale, extend your elbows back into the original plank position.
5. Remain in the position for one more round of breath, maintaining its proper alignment (the key is to engage your core—see "Belly of the Virgin").
6. Exit the pose by lowering your entire body—as a plank—slowly to the floor.

Modification: In the original plank position, lower your knees onto the floor, keeping your legs and feet elevated throughout the rest of the exercise. For further ease, the push-up may be performed against a wall, instead of the floor.

Mudra: To Invoke the Illumined Mind

Mudras are symbolic finger positions that can both invoke and evoke different states of consciousness. While their origin remains a mystery, it is known that finger gestures are considered sacred by many cultures. You can see them depicted on drawings of Hindu gods and performed as blessings during Christian church services. In the Kundalini yoga tradition every area of the hand correlates to the greater body and mind, allowing you to use your hands to access the rest of you. If you desire access to your illumined mind—before giving a talk or while writing a book—perform the *uttarabodhi mudra*, the mudra of the highest enlightenment. You will find that, apart from expanding your consciousness, performing these movements also expands the facility of your fingers and hands.

1. In a standing or seated position, place your hands in a prayer position in front of your heart.
2. Keeping the index fingers and thumbs touching each other, interlace the other fingers.
3. Point your thumbs down—they may touch your sternum—while pointing your index fingers toward the sky.
4. Close your eyes and connect with the greater wisdom you seek to elicit. Relax and breathe.

This mudra can be performed at any time, for as long as you like.

Massage: To Practice Service and Expand Nonverbal Communication

A great way to communicate your affection is by giving someone you care about a massage. You choose what type of massage—foot, neck and shoulders, back, hand, or a combination. Needless to say, the massage should be agreed upon by both parties and respect the recipient's boundaries. Whichever part you choose to connect with, consciously engage your arms, forearms, and hands in the process. As with any duality, giving comes with receiving, and as you give a good massage so, too, do you receive good strengthening for your upper extremities. If you want to add further balance to the experience for both you and your partner, employ Gemini-friendly essential oils like lavender, lemongrass, or bergamot.

Baoding Balls: To Unite Your Higher and Lower Faculties

These Chinese exercise balls are believed to have originated in Baoding, China, around the time of the Ming dynasty. Today, you can frequently find them in your local Chinatown or online. Many different exercises may be performed with these balls. Not only do these exercises increase finger and forearm strength while improving their agility, but it is also believed that they access energetic meridians that connect to organ systems throughout your body. Using these balls thereby helps you connect body, mind, and spirit. An exercise example: Rotate the balls clockwise in the palm of your hand for a few rotations and then counterclockwise for as many sets as you are comfortably able to do; the more advanced can perform these same circles with space between the two balls so they do not click as they rotate. Regardless of how many sets you do, though, you should (a) practice with each hand, and (b) pay attention to the posture of your shoulders and elbows as you manipulate the balls. Ideally, you should be sitting with relaxed shoulders and elbows, hands in your lap, palms facing up; or sit with your elbows flexed approximately ninety degrees while your forearms rest on a table or pillow. While rotating the balls, your hands may naturally tilt to garner the assistance of gravity.

Freestyle Writing: To Manifest Your Ideas

As the zodiac's messenger, the Gemini is an idea factory. He generates ideas by the dozen . . . but he is not always great at acting on them. Many brilliant books, start-ups, and devices have originated in a Gemini's mind but have not made it further. And yet, it is only when an idea is brought from internal to external reality that it can be shared, that it can serve someone other than the idea generator. Writing down your ideas is the first step to giving them greater life. So let your stream of consciousness flow, and use your hands to write (or type) for five minutes. Set an alarm to indicate when you are done (although write for longer if you choose). Whatever comes forth is fair game. In this exercise, style and grammar do not matter, nor does higher versus lower mind—the importance is simply on getting your ideas up and out! Keep what you write to reference one day. Your musings will likely bring great delight.

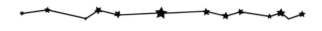

Summary

★ Your upper limbs are the regions related to Gemini. The composite arms, forearms, and hands allow you to connect to your surroundings, communicating the best of what you've got to others.

★ Gemini is the third sign of the zodiac cycle. Its energy pertains to accessing your inner illumination and imagination to deliver messages that inspire in some way, shape, or form.

★ If your brilliant Gemini nature becomes too limited in its naturally expansive scope or, conversely, is scattered everywhere, your upper limbs might experience different symptoms (e.g., muscle tension, joint instability).

★ Balance your inner Gemini through questions, exercises, and activities that focus on your upper limbs. Use them to access both sides of every dualism—be it self/other or lower/higher—and joyously juggle a world of infinite possibility.

Note

1. White House Signal Agency, "Inaugural Address, 20 January 1961," John F. Kennedy Presidential Library and Museum, accessed June 12, 2015, http://www.jfklibrary.org/Asset-Viewer/BqXIEM9F4024ntFl7SVAjA.aspx.

5

Chest of the Crab

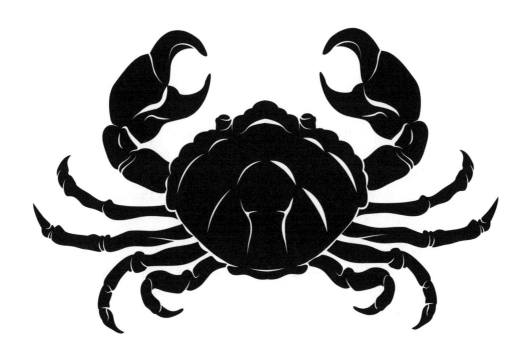

♋ CANCER

Birth date: June 21–July 22
Body region: Chest
Theme: Initiate the Cycle of
Giving and Receiving

The first quarter of the zodiac cycle—Aries, Taurus, and Gemini—was all about your birth into this world: who you are, how you express it, and the realization that you are not alone. The second quarter—Cancer, Leo, and Virgo—blooms along with summer. The self-exploration dynamic of spring has matured a bit, and the seed that started in Aries is now a plant.

Cancer commences this new phase. It is a phase that takes the self-and-other dance introduced in Gemini and sets it into a cycle. This cycle is one of giving and receiving, complementary concepts that form the foundation for most relationships in this world, starting with oneself and expanding interpersonally into home and community. Cancer not only initiates this giving-and-receiving cycle but also ensures that all aspects are well supported, balanced, and nurtured in its process.

Your Body: Chest

For the crab, her shell is, quite literally, her home. For the human Crab and all of us focusing on our Crab nature, home is where the heart is—in the chest. The chest, the body region related to the Cancer sign, is the physical representation of nourishment and nurturance, the place that our sensitive Cancer energy can turn to feel supported and protected. Starting even as a baby, the chest is considered home, as we suckle our mothers' breasts.

Through the act of breast-feeding, the child receives nourishing breast milk from his mother and, simultaneously, forges a nurturing bond with her. This iconic mother-child bond lasts a lifetime and, in all likelihood, will govern behavior during that lifetime as well. Many individuals replicate or seek the level of nurturance that was or was not given to them, acting it out in subsequent relationships. For instance, if the Cancer grew up with a mother who was unable to provide a nurturing influence, the Crab will likely repeat this dynamic in relationships where the partner is either physically or emotionally absent and does not nurture her. More than the rest of the zodiac, the Cancer nature searches for a supportive and protective home to return to.

From the musculoskeletal standpoint, the chest is that place. It features a protective cage—a rib cage—that guards the precious contents therein. Its armor is composed of twelve pairs of ribs that start in the front of your body at the breastplate (sternum), wrap around each side of the torso, and come full circle at your back, to articulate with the spine (vertebral column). And while there is a bit of

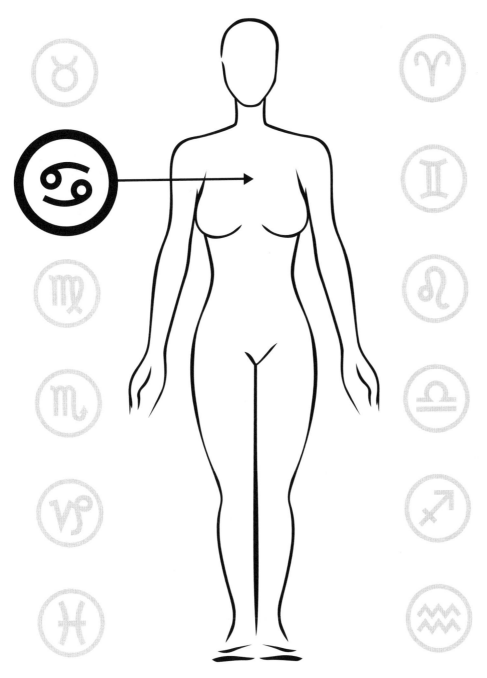

See appendix C for the skeletal structure of the chest.

mobility (the ribs elevate and depress as you inhale and exhale), the rib cage special-izes in stability. It has to, in order to maintain the safety and security of what's inside: the lungs, windpipe (trachea), food pipe (esophagus), and heart.

The presence of these respiratory and digestive structures indicates that two big biological processes happen here—respiration and digestion.

Note that the heart—despite its location within the rib cage—resides in a separate compartment than the lungs and is, along with the upper back, related to the sign of Leo (see "Heart of the Lion").

Like the breasts, both are related to Cancer's theme of nurturance. Digestion is nurturing because it is nourishing. At the physical level, you are giving your cells the food they need to develop and to support you. And then there is the context surrounding many food endeavors, which can be supportive as well—like a fine feast in the company of good friends. The term *comfort food* exists for a reason!

The respiratory tract is also considered nurturing because, like the digestive tract, it brings fuel to your cells. Its fuel, however, is in the form of oxygen that—by way of mouth, trachea, bronchi, and lungs—diffuses into your blood in order to be transported to every cell of your body. This valuable oxygen, which you received from the environment via trees and plants, is used to generate a type of energy called adenosine tri-phosphate (ATP). ATP is the energy currency of your body—it fuels every cell, allowing you to walk, breathe, and otherwise live. It is your veritable life force.

While no actual digestion occurs within the esophagus, it nonetheless plays an integral role in the process, passing food between the pharynx and stomach. Thereafter the digestion that occurs in the stomach and intestines relates to Virgo.

It's no surprise, then, that breath is considered the vehicle for life force by many traditions. For instance, it is referred to as *prana* by Ayurvedic and yogic traditions and *qi* by traditional Chinese medicine. In Christianity, breath is related to an animating force, or spirit, through its thirteenth-century etymology; the word *spirit* derives from the Latin *spiritus*, meaning "soul, vigor, breath" and is also related to *spirare*, "to breathe." Likewise, the etymological origin of *inspiration* (a technical term for the inhalation of air into the lungs) refers to the influence of God or a god. The Lisan al-Arab dictionary concurs, noting that the root for *spirit/soul* is the same as the root for *breath*, connections that the Hebrew, German, and Greek roots share.

So the breath is nurturing to body and soul—but only if you take nurturing breaths. Do you receive what you need with long, full inhales and exhales? Or are you in a perpetually anxious state, taking frequent and shallow breaths? If the latter, while you can certainly subsist on suboptimal breathing, you are depriving yourself of life force at all levels. To this extent, how well you breathe can be a litmus test for how well you nurture yourself. Use the following measures to assess the quality of your breath:

1. *Rate*. Record the number of breaths you typically take in one minute. (One breath includes both an inhale and exhale.) The average respiratory rate is about twelve to sixteen times per minute.
2. *Depth*. A full breath should involve not just the chest but also distend the abdomen. Does your regular breath enter fully into your lungs or stop around your clavicles? Does your abdomen extend with each inhale, or does it remain flat?
3. *Quality*. Close your eyes, relax, and notice the natural flow of your breath, without altering it in the process. It should be smooth and continuous. Is it? Or is it irregular? Halting? Choppy?

When is the last time you took time to notice your breath? For most individuals, the answer is never, as it is a process frequently taken for granted. Not surprisingly, then, poor breath quality is the norm rather than the exception for our modern society, where many individuals forego being and breathing for a chronic state of fight-or-flight. The result is a shorter, faster, and more superficial breath cycle that resembles the "Go go go!" and "Do do do!" influences that helped shape it. The good news is that you have the ability to change the way you breathe. You can decide to take your breath off of autopilot because respiration is one of the few biological systems that operate under both involuntary and voluntary control. Which means that you can rediscover and repattern your natural breath. One that is longer, deeper, and on the whole, much more nourishing. You just have to want to give it to, and receive it for, yourself.

The Stars: Cancer

Initiate the Cycle of Giving and Receiving

To *initiate* is to commence a new project or venture with some form of catalytic or ceremonial flair. Consider, for example, the phrase *initiate launch* just moments before the blastoff of a space shuttle. Or think of the ceremonial rituals in hunter-gatherer societies that initiate adolescents into adulthood, or the sacred teachings revealed to an initiate after walking on fire for his mystery school. In terms of Cancer, initiation comes in the form of a new phase of the zodiac cycle. While the first phase was all about the self, the next phase kicks off a more meaningful relationship with we, in the form of a relationship that is sensitive to everyone's needs. This phase helps you set up a solid framework from which to address these needs; for instance, starting a healthcare-related business, going into social work, or being a stay-at-home parent.

For the sensitive Cancer Crab nature, the drive to initiate means that there are times when she has to emerge from her shell, times when she has to expose her soft underbelly to the harsh world despite all excuses to the contrary (typically a combination of childhood memories, "coulda, woulda, shouldas," and parental blame). Breaking free from past attachments and out of one's comfort zone is no easy feat for anyone—and our emotional and intuitive Cancer energy can make matters even more challenging as we move out of the familiar and into fear. For better or worse, the only way through fear is, well, through it . . . and the light at the end of the tunnel heralds the next phase of growth. So while the hard crab shell provides a wonderful safe haven, if a person never ventures out, it becomes a hideaway instead of a supportive hearth.

Cancer's struggle between the inner and the outer is a vital component of life. Everyone needs time in their shell to shore up resources, lick wounds, amass energy for growth, and otherwise incubate free from the world. Similarly, there is a need to connect with others, experience a greater milieu, and give the resources you amassed back to it . . . until it is time to return to the shell once again. The key for the Crab is to not get stuck either inside her shell (in a dependent, self-pitying, vulnerable state), or outside of it (giving, nurturing, sacrificing). Instead, she is here to teach us all that we must find the balance between self-care and caring for others. In this way, the Cancer initiates a cycle between the two.

A cycle is a set of events or actions that happen again and again in the same order, like seasonal cycles or economic ones. Do not be fooled, however, into thinking that "same order" means "same thing." For instance, four seasons comprise one cycle, starting with spring, ending with winter, and beginning with spring again. That said, although the seasons are conceptually the same, in reality they are not. Sure, each spring entails similar components, like budding leaves on trees. But the actual leaves that bud each year are entirely different than the ones the year before, no blade of grass is the same, and neither are you. From one spring to the next, you are a different person, from your thoughts and emotions down to many cells in your body.

Without your lifting a finger, your biochemical cycles abound! Sure, you can momentarily halt your respiratory cycle by holding your breath, but your circadian cycle is always in motion, governing your twenty-four-hour physiologic processes, as is your cardiac cycle (which generates a heartbeat), urea cycle (which helps the liver detoxify your blood), and many more.

Cycles give us the chance to learn from the past—past thoughts, emotions, actions, and situations. Think about where you were one year ago. Are you able to recognize similar circumstances, patterns, or lessons in your life? If so, are you able to view them now from a different perspective? Whether you are aware of it or not, no cycle leaves you unchanged. You inevitably transformed from who you were to who you are at this very moment—and you have the opportunity to do it again. Every cycle is, in effect, a form of death and rebirth, an ebb and flow of giving and receiving that befits the compassionate nature of the zodiac sign it serves and is yours to recognize and take responsibility for within this lifetime.

Cycles start at one place and take you to another at both physical and metaphysical levels. Take, for instance, the hero's cycle (a.k.a., the hero's journey home). It occurs when a hero, like Homer's King Odysseus, ventures from his homeland and into another realm. Along the way, he encounters trials and tribulations of every ilk—from Cyclopses to sirens—that require great strength of force and will. The hero is thus transformed and returns from his adventure with new power and knowledge to share. At the more quotidian level, even the most mundane workout provides a salient example: after jogging around a track for one or more revolutions, your body ends in a different (likely fatigued but stronger) physical state from whence it began, and your thoughts and emotions are likewise transformed. Accordingly, the colloquial guidance for overcoming some form of physical or psychic stress is to run it off; you start your run in one state of body and mind, and you return in another.

The power of the cycle—whether it takes you to the island of the Cyclops or the local high school track—comes from an overarching process that encompasses

In addition to the many internal cycles affecting your body are external ones. For instance, as you read this text, the world is spinning on its axis creating the day-night cycle, while orbiting the sun in an annual cycle, while revolving (along with our solar system) around the center of the Milky Way galaxy every 225 million years. Yes, even our galaxy cycles.

The cycle of life was a recurring theme in the work of Cancer artist Gustav Klimt. In *The Three Ages of Woman* (1905), for example, the three female figures represent stages in the cycle, expressed through a child, mother, and older woman.

elements seemingly at odds. If you read the chapter "Hands of the Twins," you will recall that the Gemini superpower is to see not *or* but *and*—good and bad, right and wrong, heaven and earth. Our Cancer nature helps us further understand that these dual elements not only exist but also operate in tandem. One, in fact, leads to the other. Good and bad, right and wrong—these qualities are not necessarily opposed, nor are they even two sides of the same coin; they are two points on the same cycle.

Ebb and flow is a term typically attributed to the ocean's tides, which cycle between low (ebb) and high (flow). Tides are governed by the moon's cycles, as is the molting of crabs, which occurs with the high tides associated with the full moon. The moon also governs the zodiac Crab, Cancer, as ruling planet of the water sign. Needless to say, the moon's cycles provide countless opportunities to slough off the old and reveal the new.

Take, for example, the Cancer-related cycle of giving and receiving. In our society we place a positive emphasis on giving; good givers are deemed to be good people. Receivers, on the other hand, may be seen as selfish. And yet, if everyone were only giving, who would be available to receive? One synonym of the verb *receive* is welcome, which refers to accepting in a gracious and inviting manner. When receiving from the heart, the receiver gives great satisfaction to the giver, who then finds herself receiving through the very gift she was giving. Whew! So giving turns into receiving, receiving into giving, and suddenly there is no dichotomy between the two. There are no more discrete points but just the cycle itself.

One of the benefits of this giving-and-receiving cycle is a cared-for inner Cancer—a dynamic exchange that provides nurturance for you as well as others. It's a way for you to feel whole and wholly supported, as well as a means to enable others to do the same . . . just as long as the intent behind and execution of the exchange is legit. Because of giving's status in society, it can be easy to give (even unintentionally) as a means of validating self-worth, establishing control, or avoiding intimacy. In these circumstances, the act then becomes a false cycle of self-support as you give and give and give in search of something greater that you never seem to receive. When this happens, you are actually externalizing your sense of support, and it is an indication you need to turn inward and find nourishment within your own shell.

The natural cycle of giving and receiving should be evenly balanced. The concept "what goes around comes around" is found throughout time, space, and scripture, from Buddhist doctrines concerning karma to the New Testament's "Give, and it will be given to you" (Luke 6:38). Even the nineteenth-century robber-baron-cum-philanthropist John D. Rockefeller Sr. wrote: "I believe it is every man's religious duty to get all he can honestly and to give all he can."[1] And indeed, this Cancer lived both aspects equally. While the way he got "all he can" remains controversial, his tremendous receiving was balanced by tremendous giving. By his death, Rockefeller had donated nearly half of his billion-dollar fortune to the establishment of medical centers, universities, churches, and art foundations that still provide for society today.

Certainly, money is far from the only commodity that one can give and receive. Pretty much anything fits the bill because it is not so much what is given as how. This is why giving a loving smile can be as great a gift, or better, than new china. Because the important part is the heart with which it is given (even to yourself!). And received. So whether the gift is a smile or a set of plates or whatever, what is really being given and received is some form of love. Which, at the end of the day, is what makes the cycle nurturing for everyone.

Lessons

It is not easy to truly give, and oftentimes it's even harder to receive. Being open to someone else's offering presupposes vulnerability; it creates a space in which you allow another individual to actually affect you. What if she makes you feel a certain way? What if you cry? The questions themselves can be sufficiently scary, let alone the journey to find the answer. But if you are not journeying on the cycle of life, you are standing still on it. And if you stand still for too long, you run the risk of your wheel becoming stuck. Stuck somewhere in the netherworld between giving and receiving, which is a surefire recipe for never feeling fully nurtured.

So Cancer teaches us to learn to better receive, in order to better give . . . to ourselves, first and foremost. The entire Cancer vibe is one of nurturing, and it is of utmost importance that the Crab in you feels internally cared for in order to then help you externally direct her empathetic energy to family, friends, and community. But the vulnerability implicit in receiving help or care is a Cancer soft spot, making the Crab retreat back into her shell many times lest her sensitive nature be exploited or exposed.

This holds true even when she is the one giving herself the gift! The resistance with which our Cancer energy receives from others is merely a reflection of our inability to receive graciously from ourselves. Self-gifting in its highest form is self-love, self-care, and the Cancer is here to create that space. The cherry on top? The better able you are to meet your own needs, the better you will be at meeting the needs of others. If you are unable to meet your own needs, then your Cancer nature may get permanently stuck retreating inside her shell, burying her feelings with "why me?" type concerns that blame outside circumstances for her stuck state.

Physical manifestations of an internalized Cancer energy may include:

★ Sensation of chest tightness
★ Sunken or slumped chest
★ Kyphotic posture
★ Shortness of breath
★ Rib irritation or inflammation
★ Other: Respiratory dis-ease, esophageal dis-ease, breast lumps (e.g., cysts, fibroids)

In contrast to being internal, the Cancer—in trying to fill her shell with love and nurturing—might turn to everyone and everything else instead. Emotionally charged, she might focus on "him, her, or them" as the source of her problems and solutions. Once you relinquish your own power in the giving-and-receiving cycle, your Cancer energy then becomes an unwitting victim, and your emotions might flow without bounds as you fail to realize that the cycle is yours to turn, and no one else's.

Physical manifestations of an externalized Cancer energy may include:

★ Rib injuries (e.g., dislocation, separation)
★ Aching chest
★ Sunken or slumped chest
★ Other: Respiratory dis-ease, excess phlegm, emotional eating, heartburn, breast lumps (e.g. cysts, fibroids)

How nurturing is your chest? Whether it feels internalized, externalized, or somewhere in between, the key is listening to your body and giving it what it needs. To stretch a tight chest or strengthen a weak one, awaken your inner Cancer with the questions and exercises that follow.

Your Body and the Stars

The following will serve as your personal guide to embodying the story of the Cancer stars. Use them to initiate a new cycle of giving and receiving.

Questions

★ What do you consider to be your personal shell, the place that you find most nurturing (bedroom, beach, meditation)? What motivates you to enter your shell? What motivates you to emerge from it?

★ What do you need to give yourself to feel secure, satisfied, and supported? What do you need to receive from others to feel secure, satisfied, and supported?

★ How well do you give to yourself? To others? How well do you receive from yourself? From others?

★ What perceptions and behaviors might prevent you from giving graciously? Receiving graciously?

★ What connection do you notice between your breath and how nurtured (or not) you feel? Are you calm with a relaxed breath or hyper with a quick one?

Exercises

The Global Breath: To Give and Receive through Breath

When you inhale, you receive oxygen from the environment that gives your cells what they need. When you exhale, you give what you no longer need (carbon dioxide) back to the environment so that it receives what it needs. In this way, the cycle of breath emulates the cycle of giving and receiving—so make every breath a good one! Repattern proper respiration with the global breath, which reminds your chest how to facilitate a nourishing breath:

1. Find a calm and comfortable location to lie flat on the floor, legs extended.
2. Place your hands on your chest (in the midline, below the collarbones), one on top of the other. Breathe deeply and slowly, feeling the *anterior* expansion of your chest as it rises up and into your hands with each inhale. Repeat five times.

2. Elongate your arms by your side, with your palms flat on the floor. Breathe deeply and slowly, feeling the *posterior* expansion of your chest as your upper back presses into the ground with each inhale. Repeat five times.

4. Place one hand on each side of your rib cage (it's usually comfortable to place your hands below the level of your breasts, with fingers pointing inward). Breathe deeply and slowly, feeling how each side of your rib cage moves *laterally* (out to the side) into each of your hands, expanding so that your hands move farther apart from each other on each inhale. Repeat five times.

5. The global breath: Time to put it all together! Place your hands alongside your body, palms flat on the floor. Breathe deeply and slowly, feeling how your rib cage expands anteriorly, posteriorly, and laterally all at the same time (like a balloon), each time you inhale. Repeat five times.

As indicated by the above steps, the rib cage expands in many directions with each inhale: anteriorly, posteriorly, laterally. That is why there are so many muscles on and between your ribs—to move them! Some of the directions will be easier for you than others, which is natural. No need to judge, just observe. Practicing this exercise will help you expand your rib cage in a more balanced manner. And apart from repatterning breath, you can also use the global breath's calming effect as a tool for relaxation, improved mental focus, and increased energy. Note that the first time will take the longest in order to learn the instructions. Once you have practiced them, you can perform this sequence in about five minutes, although it is highly recommended not to rush.

Upward-Facing Dog: To Emerge from Your Shell

While the Cancer loves being warm and cozy inside her home, there are times when she must emerge. How else can she teach others the importance of balanced care? That said, it is far easier for the Crab to stay in than out (where all the predators are). Use this pose to help you come—and stay—out of your shell with a strong and open chest. When you are able to expose yourself, you need not fear others exposing you.

1. Lie on your belly on the floor. Your legs are fully extended with the tops of your feet on the floor. Your elbows are bent along your sides, and your palms are flat on the floor directly below each shoulder.

2. Press your hands equally into the floor as you straighten your arms. Lift your torso so that it arches up. Your head and neck should follow this arch, so that your gaze is up and out (but your neck is not compressed). Simultaneously, press the tops of your feet into the floor to help you lift your legs up a few inches. At this point, only your palms and feet are touching the floor.

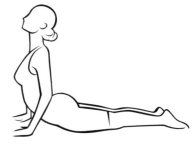

3. While in the pose, keep your thighs turned slightly inward and the arms rotated slightly outward so that the elbow creases face forward. Maintain shoulders that are down and back. Relax your lower back. Unclench your buttocks.

4. Breathe into the pose for ten rounds of inhalations and exhalations before slowly lowering yourself back to the ground.

If you want to decrease the intensity of the pose, honor Cancer compassion and increase your level of comfort by maintaining slightly bent elbows.

Kundalini Chest Opener: To Initiate Your Own Cycles

When a king crab molts, it grows out of its old shell and into a new one. The process starts a day before the actual molting, when the crab absorbs seawater that helps expand the old shell, which then starts coming apart at the seams. Followed by about fifteen minutes of pulling and pushing, kicking and yanking, the crab emerges from its old home ensconced in the new. It is a cycle of reincarnation that occurs about twenty times in its lifetime. And it can in yours too. This Kundalini practice, known as "easy pose with upper spinal flex," is a great way to intentionally enter the cycle and maintain its flow so you do not get stuck.

1. Sit in a comfortable position on the floor, with your legs crossed at the ankles. Extend your crossed ankles as far in front of you as needed to sit up straight. If necessary to enter into or maintain a proper seat, place cushions under your sitting bones.

2. Grasp your ankles firmly with your hands, keeping the elbows straight.

3. Maintaining straight elbows, arch your chest forward so it extends in front of your arms, and then curve it back behind your arms. This is one

round. Practice this movement for five rounds, keeping your chin parallel to the ground, so that your head remains level and does not move as your spine does.

4. For the next few rounds, every time your chest moves forward, inhale. Every time your chest moves backward, exhale. Keep your attention on the chest as the region of your body that is initiating the movement. The movements should be fast and vigorous yet flowing.

5. Once you feel you have found the flow, perform thirty rounds with the coordinated breath.

Once you have the rhythm in the movement, and you cycle back and forth with ease, play around with your breath. Instead of adding the breath to each movement, see if you can initiate the movement through the breath. This version will likely be more challenging, but it is equally rewarding.

Side Lying Twist: For Self-Care and Nurturing

As mentioned earlier, modern humans are well entrenched in the nervous system's sympathetic response, colloquially known as fight-or-flight. Checking off your list of to-dos as you dart from home to work to the gym to the supermarket and back home again keeps your sympathetic nervous system activated. This part of your physiology, however, is best adapted for running away from a lion, not maintaining a long-term state of alert. It is balanced by the parasympathetic system's rest-and-digest function, which allows you to breathe deeply, eat heartily, and digest thoroughly. In other words, the part of you that is all about being versus doing. The part of you that is nurturer versus achiever. Allow yourself to nurture yourself as you relax in this chest-opening twist:

1. Lie on your back with your knees bent and feet flat on the floor. Extend your arms into a *T* formation on either side of you with the palms facing up; allow the extension to flow all the way through your fingers.

2. Rotate your knees to the right on an exhale, keeping your left shoulder, arm, and hand firmly on the floor. Only rotate them so far as you are able to maintain the left shoulder-arm-hand on the floor. Try to keep your knees at an angle perpendicular to your torso. If your knees do not reach the floor, place a block beneath them for support.

3. Turn your head gently to the left, in the opposite direction your knees are pointing. Remain in this position for ten deep breaths.

4. Reverse sides by rotating your knees back to center and then to the left. Your torso remains flat on the ground. Make sure to keep the right shoulder, arm, and hand on the floor as the knees rotate left. Once the knees are in their final position (using a block if needed), rotate your head gently to the right. Remain in this position for ten deep breaths.

5. To exit the position, return your head and knees to center. Pause for a moment to enjoy your relaxed and open state before arising.

You Time: To Prioritize Self-Care

The prior exercise—the side lying twist—opened you into nurturing. With this exercise, it is time to take your deeper appreciation of self-care and prioritize it in your daily life. *It* can be any activity you consider nurturing—reading a good book, knitting, cooking, exercising, etc. The kicker is to commit to whatever it is with a good plan that patterns some healthy new habits into your day:

1. *Awareness.* Make three lists to identify (1) what nurtures you in your *ideal* lifestyle, (2) how nurturing habits exist in your *actual* healthy lifestyle, and (3) *obstacles* that exist between the two. For instance, if reading a book at bedtime is nurturing, notice that even though you want to do it nightly (ideal), you only do it once a month (actual) because of late-night emailing (obstacle).

2. *Commitment.* Choose one item from your *ideal* list that you want to—and can—do. Take the first step toward your desired lifestyle change by writing it down, recording a video, telling a coworker, or otherwise making yourself accountable.

3. *Plan.* To follow through on your commitment, create a plan that meets you where you are. It does not matter if your plan commits you to something once a week versus five times a week; what matters is that it is easily doable. Start small, and as the results speak for themselves, your health practice will naturally grow.

4. *Support.* Ask loved ones for their help implementing your plan. With what aspect can they best support you? Be as specific as possible. You might be surprised to find that once you clearly ask for their support, you will receive it.

Compliment: To Receive with Gratitude and Grace

This exercise speaks for itself . . . and yet is likely harder than you think. Find out why by doing it!

* *Part I:* Think of one thing that you are or that you do very well. For instance, you might be generous or great at knitting. It should be something that you already feel good about. Look in the mirror—maintaining eye contact—and compliment yourself with some version of: "I am [insert chosen word]! And that's awesome. In fact, I'm awesome." Smile as, and after, you say it. Pause for a moment and allow yourself to feel good.
* *Part II:* The next time someone compliments you—regardless of its magnitude or your belief in its validity—receive it as wholeheartedly as you did in part I. Respond with a genuine smile and words that show gratitude instead of disclaimers, explanations, mitigations, or the word "but."
* *Part III:* Give someone a compliment. It does not matter if it is a friend, a coworker, or a stranger—let the moment inspire you. No need to plan in advance. As soon as you see someone you think looks great in her outfit, or did a good job at work, or made a great meal, tell her so. Say it straight, simple, and with a smile. Notice how she reacts, and how it makes you feel, regardless of her response.

Summary

* Your chest is the region related to Cancer. Encasing structures that allow you to literally and figuratively take a deep breath, your personal treasure chest represents nurturance and nourishment.
* Cancer is the fourth sign of the zodiac cycle. Its energy pertains to the gifts of giving and receiving joined in a cycle that is replenishing for both yourself and others.
* If your sensitive Cancer nature withdraws too readily into its shell or exposes itself too often, your chest might experience different symptoms (e.g., shallow breath, chest tightness).

★ Balance your inner Cancer through questions, exercises, and activities that focus on your chest. Use them to delve deeper into the giving-receiving cycle, remembering that self-nurturing is necessary to nurture others best.

Note

1. Rockefeller Family & Associates, "John D. Rockefeller 1839–1937," Rockefeller Archive Center, September 1997, http://www.rockarch.org/bio/jdrsr.php.

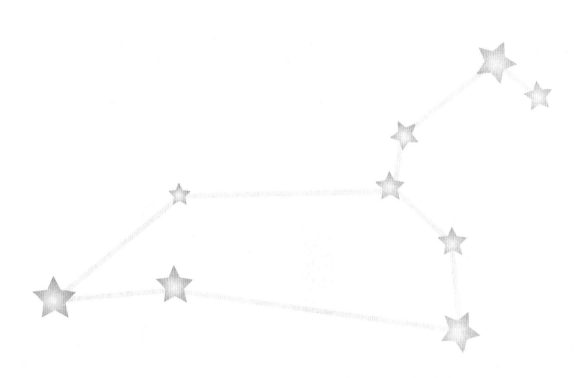

6

Heart of the Lion

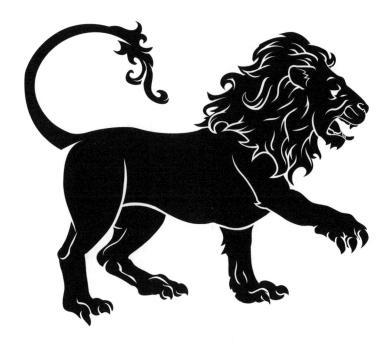

♌ LEO

Birth date: July 23–August 22
Body region: Heart, Upper Back
Theme: Shine the Light of Your Heart

The prior sign, Cancer, brings us into our body's torso, a journey that Leo continues as it dives deep into the heart—a heart that represents courage, devotion, generosity, and most poignantly, love. And it is love—primarily in the form of self-love—that the Lion is here to give, receive, and shine. His constellation possesses one of the brightest stars in the night sky (Regulus), a star that reflects exactly what the Leo is here to do: shine the light of his heart on everyone and everything around.

Your Body: Heart and Upper Back

The heart and upper back are the body regions related to the Lion. Anatomically speaking, your heart is a vital organ that pumps blood through your vessels. This blood provides oxygen and nutrients to all the cells in your body while simultaneously removing their waste (like carbon dioxide). Without this circulation, your brain would perish within four to six minutes; bone, skin, and tendons would hold out longer, but only up to twelve hours. All in all, a pretty big job for only ten ounces of muscle.

For about 2,160 years, the star Regulus has been an integral part of the Leo zodiac sign. That said, at the end of 2011, Regulus moved into the sign of Virgo, where it will stay for another 2,160 years before moving into Libra. Note, however, that the star remains in the Leo constellation. These changes are related to the apparent motion of the constellations and stars forward through the zodiac signs.

Your cardiac muscle is located near the center of your rib cage, between your lungs. While in the midst of the lungs, the heart is separated from them by the pericardium, a very thin sac that enfolds, anchors, and protects it. Physically separated from the lungs, it is also energetically separate, as astrology associates the heart with the upper back of Leo, versus Cancer's region of the chest. Note, however, that the chest and upper back are really just two sides of the same coin, with the chest correlated to the anterior rib cage and the upper back to the posterior. Together, they provide a 360-degree container for the heart, but again, astrology associates the upper back with the organ.

The upper back is made up of your thoracic vertebrae—the bones of your spine that attach to your ribs. These twelve vertebral bones reside between the neck (cervical spine) and lower back (lumbar spine). The back may be commonly considered to comprise three parts—upper, middle, and lower—or two—upper and lower. In either case, "upper and middle" or "upper" refers to the region delineated by the thoracic spine. The lower back is defined by the lumbar spine (see chapter 8: "Back

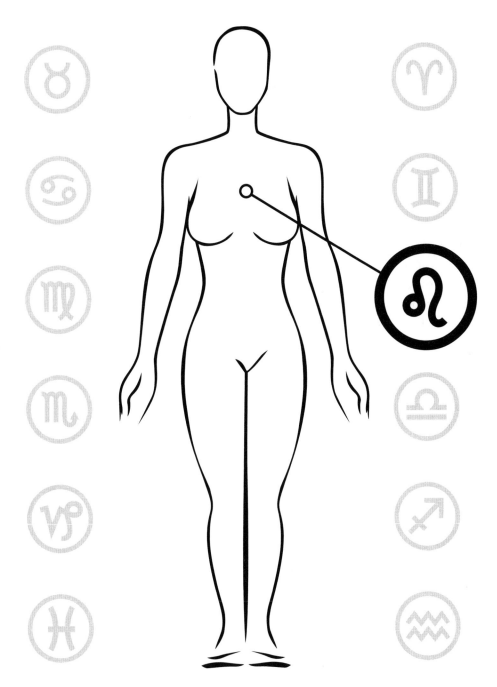

See appendix C for the skeletal structure of the upper back.

of the Scales"). Whereas the neck and lower back are designed to provide mobility, the upper back excels in strength and stability. It is part of what maintains your torso erect. Additionally, because the thoracic vertebrae connect with the ribs, the upper back helps protect the organs within the chest cavity, like the heart.

The upper back may be readily noticed in our society when it curves more than it should due to improper posture layered on top of genetic predisposition. This excessive curvature of the thoracic spine is called *kyphosis* and is perceived as stooped shoulders along with a rounding of the upper back. You might be sitting in this position now, as you read this book, or while you sit hunched over your computer. In this position, your upper back is out of alignment and your heart center hidden. Kyphosis withdraws the region of your heart from its center and toward the back of your body, like a lion retreating into its cave. This withdrawal, or excessive flexion of the thoracic spine, is a fear-based posture; it is an evolutionary mechanism that, in the face of threat, like a lion attack, is designed to protect your vital organs. But you are not built to maintain this fear-based posture throughout the day. You are meant to stand upright, with shoulders back and heart centered.

For many of us, hiding our hearts has been patterned over so many years that it feels scary to stick it out . . . even if sticking it out simply returns your thorax to its natural alignment and stability. This position may be more expansive than what you are used to, more exposed. Which means that standing with your heart open, you may feel vulnerable—vulnerable to other people judging you. But no one has the power to make you feel a certain way unless you give it to them. So if you feel hurt, angered, or otherwise charged by another's comments, it may be because they touch upon a part of you that you have not fully accepted—the shadows within, which you are judging (perhaps unwittingly) too. These shadows are why your Leo might not want to look inside. Instead, he might perceive that it is easier to hide the heart altogether, or cover it up with false confidence and pride. And so he may paradoxically puff out his chest to look big in order to compensate for feeling small. Perhaps the most iconic depiction of this stance is through the portraits of Leo Emperor Napoleon Bonaparte, and his eponymously named complex.

 The Napoleon complex is a popular term for the belief that men who are short in stature may compensate with extreme drive, narcissism, and megalomania. That said, while Emperor Napoleon was not the tallest man, some historians believe that he was actually average height in France at the time but looked small in portraits because he was depicted surrounded by large guards.

How do you carry your heart center? Look at your upper back to find out:

1. Stand in front of a mirror and turn sideways for a profile reflection. Stand as you normally would if you were not paying attention to your posture (no cheating!). Rotating your head as minimally as possible, look toward the mirror and observe the prominence—or not—of the curve of your upper back.

2. Exaggerate the natural C curve of your upper back so that your shoulders round forward. In this position, your head and neck will come forward and down as well. Now, repeat the Leo motto: "Here I am!" Notice how it feels and sounds.

3. Stand up in what you would consider your ideal alignment. Your head should stack on top of your heart, your heart on top of your hips, your hips over your knees, and your knees over your feet. It should feel as if your entire body is dangling in one straight line from a string. Now, repeat the Leo motto: "Here I am!" Notice how it feels and sounds.

Chances are that your natural stance (step 1) falls somewhere between the kyphotic posture (step 2) and your ideal one (step 3). If this is the case, then you are hiding your heart as you move throughout the day. You are subsequently foregoing the full extent of strength and stability that your upper back would otherwise impart to the rest of your self, which is why it was likely harder to vocalize in step 2. The good news is that you always have the ability to access this region more and more. You have the opportunity, every day, to straighten your spine, expand into your heart and confidently state, "I am lion, hear me roar!"

The Stars: Leo

Shine the Light of Your Heart

The sun is the center of our solar system. Its gravitational pull draws eight planets, at least five dwarf planets, tens of thousands of asteroids, and millions of comets around it. Whether we're considering a planet that orbits it, a plant that grows toward it, an ancient who worshipped it, or a beachgoer who basks in it, the sun commands attention. People are drawn to light. And the sun is, as far as our solar system is concerned, the brightest light. You feel its power as heat on your skin and see it as light with your eyes. From planets to people, it illumines everyone and everything.

Its luminous quality exemplifies the sign of Leo, whose ruling planet is, indeed, the sun—the sun-lion relationship is a long-standing one, evidenced throughout Persian, Semitic, and ancient Egyptian lore. So the Leo energy represents the shine that the sun possesses, present and resplendent within us all. To *shine* means to give forth light. Leo does so by standing tall, confident in who he is and in his desire to display his glory to the world at large. It is as if he has been rehearsing behind the scenes during the past five zodiac signs and is now ready to command center stage. The Leo energy knows who he is and what he is good at, and he is so comfortable in his own skin that he wants to show it off to anyone around. And like the sun, the energy that Leo shines is immense—so much so that when he shines, he not only lights up himself, but he also illumines others. This sunny nature will fawn on them, encourage them, and help them cultivate their shininess too, just as long as our inner Leo, like the sun in times past, is revered in return.

If our inner Leo does not receive what he perceives as his proper due, then watch out for solar flares! Just as the sun may abruptly emit a high-intensity ray, the Lion can likewise erupt if he does not get what he wants. He wants—nay, feels entitled to—the praise, adornment, and adulation that accompany center stage. With a boastful roar, this volatile king—of the jungle and beyond—demands his own way. Or else. Think of former world rulers like Napoleon, Mussolini, and Castro. They were all Leos whose megalomania played out very dramatically on the world stage, as they demanded the respect and admiration of militaries and nations. And while supporters were rewarded with the highest rank, if the leader's desired level of subservience was not received—or if his belief system was opposed—retaliation was swift and decisive. Such is the harmful hubris of the Leo who is so blinded by his light that he fails to see his shadow.

In addition to the sun, the lion is traditionally associated with royalty as the king of beasts. Lions may therefore be seen on many a flag, crest, and coat of arms from Britain to Sri Lanka, Iran, Australia, and beyond. Even the Leo constellation is closely associated with royalty, as the name of its brightest star, Regulus, means "little king." This star, located at the bottom of the celestial lion's mane, shines 140 times as brightly as our sun.

Your inner light serves the same purpose as the sun—it helps you see. It is an internal flame that shines with the brightness of who you are at your healthiest, happiest, highest self. And it radiates not only your personal truth, but also the greater truth embodied within the light of the universe. It is the part of you that feels divine, special, magical. Like everything is just as it needs to be and is a-okay. It is comparable to being in the zone, a space in which time ceases to exist—as do worries, fears, and concerns. If you believe in it, you might call this light your spirit or soul. And when you are ensconced in it, you may say that you are en-light-ened.

Yes, your inner light is ribbons and rainbows and everything nice. However, it is also the source of your deepest, darkest shadows. A shadow is the area where light cannot reach due to obstruction. When you are outside, walking down the street in the afternoon, that obstruction is you—blocking the light en route from sun to cement—which is why you cast a shadow. Internally, that obstruction is the part of you known as your dark side, the part of you that is less than pure light. Your personal bumps in the road that represent traits you have not accepted, refuse to see, or otherwise do not like, even if you do not know exactly what they are or how they got there.

It is typically a challenge to accept the less-than-perfect parts of yourself. It is much easier to walk down the road with your face toward the sun, pretending that your shadow does not exist. As they say, ignorance is bliss. But one of the tasks of Leo is to use his light to acknowledge his dark—otherwise, our Leo nature can get out of whack, as illustrated by the rulers mentioned above. And it is fitting that none other than the Leo psychotherapist Carl Jung was the one to shed light on this subject with his shadow theory. "The shadow," wrote Jung, "is that hidden, repressed, for the most part inferior and guilt-laden personality whose ultimate ramifications reach back into the realm of our animal ancestors and so comprise the whole historical aspect of the unconscious."[1] It is a part of your primordial self, a darkness that is as entrenched in you as is the light. To deny your shadow is to deny an aspect of yourself. Believe it or not, even the parts that you do not like, that you consider dark, have served their purpose in helping you arrive exactly where you are today (recall the lesson in Gemini, in which there is not light or dark but light and dark). These shadow aspects have had their own role to play, and the Leo is here to help you actively involve them in the game.

> The universe tells us its story mainly through light, which is emitted or absorbed by all living and nonliving things on Earth, as well as surrounding stars, planets, and galaxies. It also shows us the vast majority of the universe (96 percent) that consists of dark matter and dark energy, which we otherwise cannot see.

Engaging these deeper, darker aspects of yourself takes a lot of light (again, because it is impossible to see shadows without light)—along with a hefty dose of courage. For, after you see your shadow, your Leo bravura will help you not run from it but face it squarely in the eye. And after you face it once, your Leo will help you do so again and again as your shadow continually reappears. A shadow, like the light that forms it, may take a variety of forms; for those with Leo prominently in their chart, these forms often feature excessive pride, arrogance, and narcissism—or you might experience those if you are simply blocked in that area. Regardless of its manifestation, Leo helps you make the choice to either take personal responsibility for developing these lesser aspects of your nature or avoiding them. If you choose the former, then your Leo nature may feel victorious as he evolves both inside and out. If the latter, then he may either project his unwanted qualities onto others or be dominated by them without even realizing it. In other words, either you slay your inner beast or it slays you.

♌ In his first of twelve labors—self-inflicted punishment for killing his family—the ancient Greek hero Hercules was tasked to slay the lion of Nemea, a beast that no weapon could wound. So Hercules had to face it eye to eye and engage it hand to hand. Ultimately, Hercules slew the beast—which represented his inner shadow—and emerged victorious, wearing its coat as a mark of pride.

But take heart! For this form of your Leo nature is here to help you overcome your inner obstacles. Throughout time and culture, the heart has represented our most elevated qualities. Take the Egyptian *Book of the Dead*, which equated our hearts with our characters. At the end of our lives, we would be judged according to the weight of our hearts, against that of a feather. If our heart was lighter, we would gain access to the afterworld. If it was heavier, then we would be condemned to nonexistence. Of course, the ancient Egyptians were neither the first nor last to symbolize the heart as a gateway to the divine. Within traditional Chinese medicine, the heart houses the spirit *(shen)*, which gives elevated purpose, presence, and meaning to your life. In a phrase attributed to the Hindu Upanishads, it is similarly decreed that spirit resides in the heart: "Radiant in light, yet invisible in the secret most place of the heart, the spirit is the supreme abode wherein dwell all that move and breathe and see." And even the poster child for mind-body separation, René Descartes, believed that the heart was the source of the body's heat and one example of "the body as a machine created by the hand of God."[2]

Needless to say, throughout countless cultures the heart connects to *a lot*. Joy, courage, strength—like light itself, the heart's light can adopt myriad forms. Perhaps, though, its most famous form is love, which itself comes in a whole host of shapes and sizes. Leo energy is most connected with self-love: a state of total self-awareness and self-acceptance, an appreciation of your light *and* dark. And it is also a practice that honors your fully integrated being through aligning thoughts with actions, intent with execution. It manifests daily as choices congruent with your bio-psycho-spiritual growth and choices made without fear. Self-love, then, is what gives every Lion the courage to shine in his own way. When you feel wonderful about your shiny self, you want others to feel that same love and satisfaction for themselves.

But self-love starts within before it can radiate out—this concept is reflected in one of the most famous phrases from the New Testament's Gospel of Matthew, "Love your neighbor as yourself." That's the beauty of self-love done right—it is all about you *and* all about them. After engaging your inner Gemini, you know it is no longer one or the other, and your Cancer helped reinforce the giving-receiving exchange. So now Leo can help you embrace the purest form of self-love, one that is neither narcissism nor entitlement. Rather, it is an appreciation of who you are and what you have to give, along with taking responsibility for making it happen. You know what you need and what you deserve, and nothing less will do. And it shouldn't.

> In traditional Chinese medicine, organs represent metaphysical networks that complement their physical structures and functions. For instance, while the heart circulates blood, it also stores the *shen* (spirit, intelligence), the kidney regulates fluid levels and the body's *jing* (essence), and the lung governs respiration as well as distribution of *qi* (life force).

Lessons

Living with heart is available to everyone, from the most basic to the most advanced practitioner. And even if you feel that you are already living from a heart-centered place, your work is not done. This is because the metaphysical light that shines through the physical organ is eternal, providing an endless supply of fuel to grow and glow. Infinite in scope, it stands in contrast to the finite fuel of the mind with its continuous filtering, rationalizing, and quantifying. The mind serves a very important means of perceiving your self and your surroundings—but its means are only one of many.

The light of the heart provides another valuable means of ascertaining life, with all of its sensing, resounding, expounding, exploring, and celebrating. With the backing of your heart, your Leo energy is bound to be magnificent. When you love yourself, you feel confident to voice your opinions loudly, boldly, abundantly—in other words, to roar. Your Leo is here to channel the heart's expanse and shine it brightly through you—his human form.

And when he does, he balances the head-heart equation by reigniting the fire of the heart. In so doing, he tacitly gives permission to all those around him to do the same. Leo is the first person on an empty dance floor, the courageous soul who, with his zest, inspires the others to get up and groove.

Take heed, though. The brighter Leo shines, the more shadows will appear. So when you are really engaging your Leo, you must be ready to expose your shadows to yourself . . . before getting on stage for all others to see. Otherwise, two outcomes might occur. First, if your Leo has you concentrating only on the good and ignoring the bad and the ugly, then what you are showing off will be false—false pride, false courage, false confidence, false self-love. *False* creates a facade that's outer reflection is not backed by internal strength. When this bravado occurs, Leo might then manifest as self-centeredness, narcissism, egoism, and demandingness—imposing standards on others that are impossible to attain in order to make him feel better or superior.

Physical manifestations of a grandiose Leo nature may include:

★ Puffed-out chest
★ Held breath
★ Upper back tightness or tension
★ Limited mobility of upper back and shoulder blades
★ Other: Heart dis-ease

Or if your Leo struggles with awareness of and acceptance of his shadow, he might forego falsity for full retreat and head back into his lair, and you'll end up living smaller than who you are. After all, Leo has the power to eclipse his own light, just as the sun can be eclipsed by the moon. And just as an eclipse will eventually come to an end, Leo can certainly shine again . . . but only after the darkness is understood and integrated into the light.

Physical manifestations of a cowardly Leo nature may include:

Because the thoracic spine is inherently stable (due to the presence of the rib cage), it incurs fewer injuries and degenerative processes than the surrounding cervical and lumbar spines.

★ Sunken chest
★ Kyphotic posture
★ Upper back ache, weakness, or fatigue
★ Shallow breath
★ Other: Heart dis-ease

How expansive is your heart center? Whether it feels grandiose, cowardly, or somewhere in between, the key is listening to your body and giving it what it needs. To stretch a tight upper back or strengthen a weak one, awaken your inner Leo with the questions and exercises that follow.

Your Body and the Stars

The following will serve as your personal guide to embodying the Leo stars. Use them to shine the light of your heart.

Questions

★ When do you feel your brightest (who is present, where are you, what are you wearing, what are you doing)? What prevents you from shining?

★ How do you get in touch with your inner light?

★ How would you describe your shadow side? In what ways do these traits help you? Hinder you?

★ How do you encourage your friends, family, and colleagues to shine?

★ Do you stand with your back straight and heart open? What circumstances facilitate this alignment? In which circumstances do you find yourself with a rounded upper back and hidden heart?

Exercises

Sphinx Pose: To Strengthen Your Power

In ancient Egypt, the sphinx is a mythical creature with the body of a lion and the head of a human. It is believed to symbolize the pharaoh and his rule—one of power and reason. The lion's body represents great strength, while the human visage symbolizes intelligence and control. Reestablish your reign by getting in touch with your inner pharaoh, your noble lion. The sphinx pose will bring these parts up and out, as you open and align the entire expanse that surrounds your heart—chest, upper back, and even your shoulder blades (scapulae):

1. Lie on your belly on the floor, legs extended side by side. The tops of your feet should be flat on the floor.

2. Place your elbows under your shoulders so that your forearms rest on the floor in front of you, parallel to each other.

3. Engage your feet and reach your toes toward the wall behind you.

4. On an inhale, lift your torso up and away from the floor into a mild back extension.

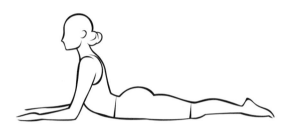

5. You are now in sphinx pose. To fine-tune the position, drop your shoulders away from your ears. Keep your forearms alive and alert all the way through your fingers. Feel your pubic bone (the front of your pelvis) push gently into the floor, while your lower back relaxes. Release your buttocks if they are clenched. Your neck should be positioned as a natural extension of your spine, not overextended. Hold for five deep breaths.

6. To exit the position, slowly lower your torso to the floor.

7. Repeat one or two more times.

Even though this pose is still, infuse it with a dynamic energy that befits the regal history and mystery of the sphinx. For instance, even though your arms and legs are not moving, keep them engaged and extended.

Camel Pose: To Open into Your Heart's Light

Camels are renowned for carrying a lot of weight. They lug bags on their backs as they traverse the desert, enduring life without water for up to six months. While this burden is physical, throughout the centuries camels have come to symbolize the endurance needed to move through metaphysical burdens as well. Friedrich Nietzsche's description of a spiritual life contains three metamorphoses, and the first is symbolized by the camel. The second stage is that of the lion. As the lion, you are no longer taxed by the weight of the world. Instead you realize *your* will upon the world. In this way you step into your own light and, in so doing, are better able to fight the dark (represented by a dragon). Use camel pose to move through your burdens and into your heart's light.

1. Kneel on the floor with your knees hip distance apart. Press your shins and the tops of your feet into the floor. Unclench your buttocks. Find a neutral position for your pelvis, so that it is neither tucked nor extended.

2. Place your palms on the back of your pelvis—one palm on each side of your spine—with fingers together and pointing down. Keep your shoulders down, away from your ears.

3. Inhale and extend your upper back, lifting and opening your heart. Your head and neck should serve as a continuation of your spine, also in a supported arch; your gaze will be up and out. (If this position is too taxing on your neck, tuck your chin in, toward your neck for great support.) While your upper torso extends, make sure that your lower back does not, and that your pelvis remains in the neutral position in which you started. Stay in this position for ten breaths.

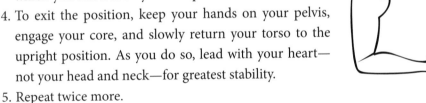

4. To exit the position, keep your hands on your pelvis, engage your core, and slowly return your torso to the upright position. As you do so, lead with your heart—not your head and neck—for greatest stability.

5. Repeat twice more.

For a greater opening, advanced practitioners may enter into the full pose by increasing the extension of the back so that the palms ultimately rest upon the soles of the feet. For all: a nice counter pose to camel pose's deep extension is the flexion in child's pose, in which you bring your buttocks back toward, and if possible, onto your heels, while laying your torso between your thighs so that your forehead rests on the ground, with arms elongated by your sides. The child, by the way, is Nietzsche's third and final stage.

Lion Pose: To Roar with Confidence

When is the last time you made a funny face? Chances are, not since you were a child, or with one. Children stick their tongues out all the time, in part because they do not care what others think—they are making the funny face because it pleases them to do so. It is an expression of who they are at that moment in time, and they do not think twice about it—because the child lives less from the head and so much more from the heart, which is a place that knows no fear. It is a shame that most adults lose this innate confidence and retreat into their lairs. After all, funny faces are just flexion and extension of facial muscles. At the physical level, that is it. But at the metaphysical level, making a funny face as an adult has so much more to do with what others think. Or rather: what you think others are thinking of you. So get out of your head and into your heart with lion pose. Harken back to your heartfelt confidence from childhood and roar!

1. Kneel on the floor, with toes curled under and your buttocks resting on your heels. Place your hands upon your thighs, with palms facing down and fingers spread wide.
2. Inhale deeply through your nose, filling up your chest and upper back with air.
3. Exhale forcefully and fully make a *ha* sound while:
    * Opening your mouth wide and sticking your tongue out and down toward your chin as far as it will go
    * Opening your eyes wide and gazing upward toward the third eye (midbrow)
    * Pressing your palms against your thighs with straight arms
4. Repeat three times, louder and more vigorously each time.

Dolphin Pose: For Strength of Heart

This pose is effective for strengthening and stabilizing the musculoskeletal structures that surround the heart. The key is to keep your back straight (not sunken), your chest broad, and your shoulder blades down and flat. Strength begets strength, so the more you practice this pose, the more easily you will be able to maintain the heart center's proper alignment both on and off the mat. In time you will notice that it becomes easier not only to stand with a strong heart but to act from one too.

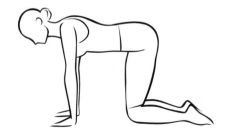

1. Start in a tabletop position on your hands and knees.

2. Lower your forearms to the floor so that your shoulders are aligned directly over your elbows. From this position, bring your palms together (forearms will angle toward the midline) and interlace your fingers. Make sure that the outer edges of the pinkie fingers are firm against the floor.

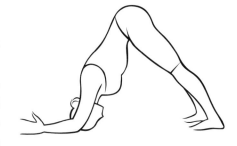

3. Pressing your forearms into the floor, curl your toes under, exhale, and extend your legs, allowing your sitting bones to rise toward the ceiling so that you are now in an upside-down V). Your feet are hip distance apart. Your head and neck should be an extension of your spine, in a straight line; your gaze falls between your mid-thighs.

4. Press your scapulae flat against your back so that your shoulders do not curve (if your shoulders still curve, slightly bend your knees). Depress your shoulder blades away from your ears. Your entire torso—from pelvis to elbows—should form one flat line.

5. Breathe for at five least slow and controlled rounds.

6. Exit the pose by releasing your knees to the floor on an exhale.

First lions, then camels, now dolphins . . . animals have the power to be great teachers if we tune in to the greater messages they bring. Whether these animal totems are found within Native American or shamanic lore, the messages are similar throughout. The dolphin, for example, represents—among many qualities—the purest form of love. Remember the *Book of the Dead* mentioned earlier in the chapter? Instead of Anubis delivering a worthy soul to the afterworld (after his heart was weighed), in some ancient Roman myths, a dolphin carried them to the Islands of the Blessed. And according to the Greeks, the dolphin is the compatriot of Apollo, the sun god and, accordingly, a god associated with Leo. So dolphin pose really has it all—a way for you to strengthen your connection to your heart at all levels.

Make a List: To Face Your Shadows

Many times, the parts we do not like in ourselves are so well hidden from our view that we project them straight onto others. For example, entitlement might be one of your hot buttons, the trait you really cannot stand in another. When you see it, you might even say to yourself, "She is so entitled! I would never act like that." Frequently, however, traits we dislike most in others represent what we dislike most in ourselves. That is why there is so much of a charge when you see it—because it is reflecting a part of you that you have yet to accept. If this is the case, then entitlement (or whatever your hot button) is likely governing your life more than you realize. Until, that is, you shed light on it and bring it into your active awareness. Once you see it you can do something about it and decide to either let it keep governing your behavior or turn the tables and become the governer. See what you have not been willing to see by shedding light on your shadows.

1. Make a list of traits you cannot stand in others. Do not censor yourself—anything that comes to mind is fair game.
2. Choose the top three traits that drive you crazy. Think of specific examples of how, when, and with whom you have encountered them.
3. For each of these traits, review to see if it is a quality that you have demonstrated in the past or present. Think of specific examples. Be honest and objective. This exercise is not about blame or self-castigation. It is simply to observe parts of yourself that you might not have observed before.
4. That's it! Awareness is the first step to overcoming your shadows and this alone will help a needed transformation occur. You may even become more aware of how these traits emerge in your daily interactions.

Next steps involve acceptance of your shadow traits and an inner responsibility for them, followed by a plan of action to allow them to evolve.

Self-Embrace: For Simple Self-Love

Love yourself. The Leo is all about abundance, and there is always more than enough love to go around. Open yourself to receiving more love, giving it, receiving it, and giving it again. Remember entering this giving-and-receiving cycle from the Cancer stage of the zodiac? Now is your time to embrace it. Literally and fully.

1. Sit up straight in a chair, with your feet flat on the floor. Close your eyes.
2. On a deep inhale, lift your heart, neck, and head and open your arms wide to both sides. This should be as expansive a position as you can make it.

3. On a deep exhale, return your torso to its neutral position, wrapping your arms around you in a self-embrace. Your head and neck will likely lower, but make sure not to cave in your chest!

4. Repeat for one minute, creating a continuous flow between the inhales and exhales. As you move, feel the love that you are opening into, receiving, and giving. Give it your own flair. This movement should be pleasurable, fun . . . and it might even make you smile.

An embrace imparts love at all levels. For instance, it is believed that, among its many benefits, a good hug releases oxytocin to promote sensations of connection and trust, activates receptors on the skin that lower blood pressure, and lowers cortisol levels to impart calm.

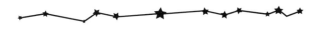

Summary

★ Your heart and upper back are the regions related to Leo. They represent your courage, love, and devotion to who you are and what you've got.

★ Leo is the fifth sign of the zodiac cycle. Its energy pertains to your inner light and being able to shine it straight from the heart (despite the shadows that result!).

★ If your Leo nature turns too self-centered or, afraid of the spotlight, retreats, your heart and upper back might experience different symptoms (e.g., muscle tightness or weakness).

★ Equilibrate your inner Leo through questions, exercises, and activities that focus on your heart and upper back. Use them to amplify your own glow and ignite others' flames.

Notes

1. Stephen A. Diamond, "Shadow," in *Encyclopedia of Psychology and Religion L–Z*, ed. David A. Leeming, et al., (New York: Springer Science+Business Media, 2010), 836.

2. René Descartes, *Discourse on Method and Meditations* (New York: Macmillan, 1960), 41.

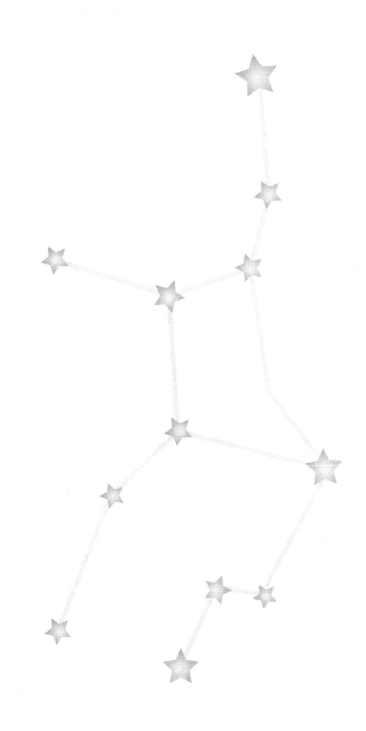

7

Belly of the Virgin

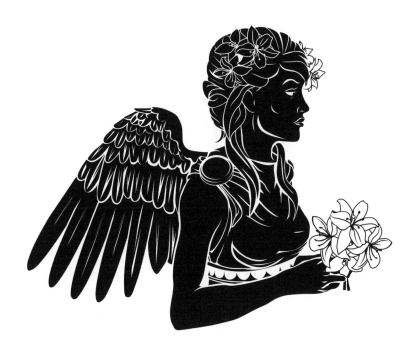

♍ VIRGO

Birth date: August 23–September 22
Body region: Abdomen
Theme: Serve with Purity of Purpose

Coming from Leo with an awareness of light and dark nature, Virgo desires to distill it, to remove any and all impurities—to tame Leo's beast. Life is no longer about her but about what she is able to give. After all, it is harvest time! The crops that came to fruition under Leo are now—with the end of summer—ready to be reaped. Ready for the grain to become bread and the grape to become wine. But first, Virgo must separate the wheat from the chaff, for she is here to serve the earth's bounty in its purest form.

Your Body: Abdomen

Are you familiar with the saying "You are what you eat?" Well, it is true. Food that you eat ultimately turns into you. It is a practical magic that occurs via absorption, a process of the small intestine, one of the organs in the abdominal region related to Virgo. Here, a walnut that began as something seemingly separate from you finishes being digested into its molecules, as protein, fat, and so on. These molecules, via your bloodstream, are then delivered to the rest of you and become, for example, parts of your hair or hormones.

> ♍ Virgo is the largest constellation of the zodiac and the second largest in the sky (after Hydra). It encompasses the autumnal equinox, the point at which the sun's ecliptic intersects the celestial equator. Astrologically, though, it is Libra that celebrates the start of autumn in the Northern Hemisphere.

Your small intestine—the facilitator of this practical magic—is only one component of your abdominal cavity. In fact, the bulk of your body's organs reside there in addition to it, including the large intestine, liver, and stomach. One of the Latin roots of *abdomen*, *abdere*, means "to hide" and, indeed, much is hidden within the abdomen. The abdomen is the region of your body that extends between the diaphragm and pelvis. While most people are aware of the abdomen's inner contents, you are more likely familiar with its outer makeup—the four sheets of muscle that comprise your abdominal wall. The most famous sheet, the rectus abdominis, is the outermost muscle that is responsible for your six-pack. Whether or not you can see it, you have a six-pack. It is part of your DNA, formed by tendinous insertions that partition the rectus abdominis muscle into six, or even eight, divisions. The transversus abdominis is the innermost muscle, a thin sheath that's entire purpose is to compress the contents within. This muscle does such an amazing job of stabilizing your insides that it forms the anterior portion of your core; two of the other abdominal muscles, the obliques, form its sides.

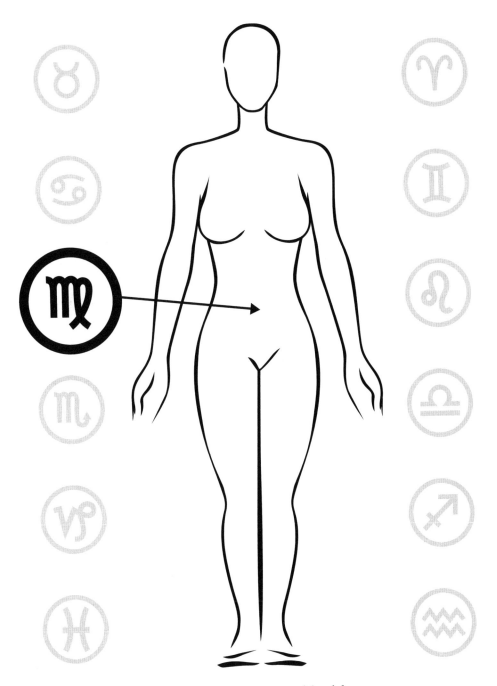

See appendix C for the structure of the abdomen.

Astrologically, the core is the container for your Virgo energy. Physically, the *core* is an old concept and a contemporary term that refers to anatomically and functionally interconnected muscles of the lower back, abdomen, and pelvis. These muscles synergistically stabilize your spine and include the diaphragm, pelvic diaphragm, abdominal wall muscles, and deep muscles of the back. Together, they help your torso maintain a protective posture in the face of destabilizing forces—like a moving train, a football tackle, or flailing limbs during dance class.

The core muscles are distinguished from other stabilizing muscles in the body due to their location, which encompasses the body's center of mass, like a corset. Our center of mass matters because the rest of our body behaves as if all of its mass were concentrated there. The center of mass is, therefore, the point around which your entire body can be balanced (think of a hanging mobile). For instance, when standing on one leg, once you locate your center, then it does not matter how you position your free leg. Whether you rest your free foot on your ankle, calf, or suspend it in the air, your overall balance will not be disturbed. It will likewise not be disturbed if your hands are on your waist or extending above you. The opposite is also true: if you are unable to locate your center, you will not be able to stand on one leg independently of where your other leg and arms are.

♍ Your gut has a mind of its own. In fact, it has an entire nervous system that contains a whopping one hundred million neurons. While it is known that this second brain oversees the physical processes of the gut (digestion, absorption, elimination) without needing input from your head's brain, it is increasingly clear that it helps regulate emotion as well.

Finding your center is no easy feat in yoga class, let alone in the rest of life, where destabilizing forces abound. Whether these forces come from a job, family pressure, or your own sense of what needs to get done, it can be easy to feel as though you've lost your center as you are pulled in many directions at once. The good news is that your center is never truly lost. Even if you cannot seem to find it, it is always there. Because it is your core! It is your inner authority, your gut instinct, so to speak. The place that knows exactly who you are and why you are here.

When you are in this place—in your purpose—you give power to the rest of you too. At the physical level, using your core as the genesis of your movements allows your arms and legs to function at their best. That is, to most efficiently serve their own purpose. And your inner Virgo is nothing if not efficient! Metaphorically speaking, when you tune in to your core, you tap into a profound fuel that is like a fire burning in your belly. It is a deep sense of your identity, worth, and power that exceeds your mind's ability, a level of analysis and exactitude of self that is part and parcel of this zodiac sign. How adept are you at accessing your core? Try this modified plank position to test it out:

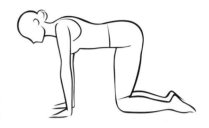

1. Start in a tabletop position on your hands and knees, with wrists under shoulders and knees under hips. Neck is neutral, with the gaze down and slightly in front of you on the floor.
2. Place your forearms on the ground, parallel to each other. Engage your core, press down through your forearms, curl your toes under, and extend your knees. You are now in the forearm plank position. Hold for sixty seconds.

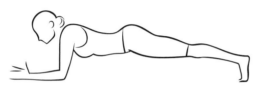

If you can complete the test—holding the pose without sinking in the shoulder or pelvic girdles, or dipping in the knees—you have good core strength. If not, your core strength needs improvement.

You can frequently observe a person's lack of purpose through her slumped stance. Her stance appears if her body is running low on energy and conviction. There is no clear center, no purpose to her form. No locus is driving her movements. Even her gaze does not intentionally land. If you try a slumped stance for yourself, you will see that is not easy to move through life like this! It is hard to harness your body's energy when it is unwittingly dispersed throughout. And yet, you have only one body. And to take the best care of it—and you—its movements should not occur by happenstance but with purpose. At any given point, be aware of how your skeletal frame is positioned in space—and why. It starts with finding your center, your core.

The Stars: Virgo

Serve with Purity of Purpose

To be of service is to provide assistance, to act helpfully. And you get to decide how, for there are no specifications or restrictions on what constitutes the service you provide. As long as you can conceive of and give a service, it exists—from a smile to a sandwich to a sermon. Its magic is in the how—which is what distinguishes a service from, let's say, a transaction. The how is the way in which the smile or sandwich is given—the intent, integrity, honesty, and heart (or not)—behind it. Service appears as a theme many times throughout the zodiac cycle, and at the Virgo stage, service is not service without these components.

These components define not just what you give but also the way in which you give, rendering the nature of the server and her service inseparable. Take the farmer, for example, who sells the corn at your local market. The attention and diligence with which she cultivated her crop is likewise apparent in the way in which she sells it at her tent. She might give you a free sample to taste how good it is, offer you ideas for the leftover cob, or just look you in the eye and smile. She is appealing not to the mind of her customer but to the heart. Which is why this purchasing experience is likely very different than a transaction involving a similar piece of corn in a city supermarket.

The concept of service may now be understood at a deeper level. Recall that it was introduced under Gemini's watch (see chapter 4: "Hands of the Twins"). His service—in the form of innovative ideas and messages—needed to reach a broader audience. It was not enough for the message to appeal to just the Gemini's mind; it also had to benefit others. Now with Virgo, service finds its roots not with the server or served but in the service itself. That is why the exchange at your local market is likely more fulfilling than at the supermarket—the farmers market stand exists not just for the sake of the seller or purchaser but for the corn too. For the corn is not just corn but a representation of earth, nature, sustenance, community, and hard work. So the Virgo aspect of the farmer plants, grows, harvests, and otherwise serves the corn because she sees herself as a conduit for the corn and everything it represents. She is simply providing a way for the produce to achieve its highest good, which allows her to achieve *her* highest good as well. Whether food, jewelry, or therapy, devotion to service can take many forms, all of which are embodied in Virgo's constellation of the virgin maiden.

The archetype of the virgin maiden has been heralded through time and space—Shala was the Sumerian embodiment, Isis took shape in ancient Egypt, Demeter in ancient Greece, the Vestal Virgins in Rome, and the Virgin Mary in the Middle Ages. More recently was the Virgo Mother Teresa, who vowed, through the

♍ The Vestal Virgins were female priestesses responsible for maintaining the ancient city's sacred fire. As long as it burned, the city would endure. Fittingly, their namesake is Vesta, the Roman goddess of fire and, more recently, the name of the brightest asteroid visible from Earth.

Order of the Missionaries of Charity, to give "wholehearted free service to the poorest of the poor." Of course, the moniker "virgin maiden" is not to be taken literally: as maidens, these women represent those who serve the fruits of the earth to the people of the earth. And as virgins, their service was considered modest, undefiled, and pure.

According to the ancient Greek philosopher Plato, the world is made up of forms—or properties—that are pure in and of themselves. Take, for example the property of roundedness, such as in baseballs, marbles, oranges, wheels, the general shape of planet Earth, etc. But while roundedness characterizes each of these things, it is nonetheless its own entity, as are size, shape, weight, and color. Even if all balls and marbles were destroyed, the concept of roundedness would remain. It stands as its own quality. Certainly, roundedness can mix with other elements like weight or color in order to create a more complex entity like an orange or a ball, but by itself it is what it is. Just pure roundedness. Never changing. Eternal.

Needless to say, pure roundedness is hard to find. You do not see it rolling down the street. It needs other characteristics—like dimension—to tangibly exist. But as soon as it merges with other characteristics, its purity is diluted. So, while purity is a state—a freedom from anything that contaminates—it is also a quest. A quest to achieve the absolute essence of whatever a thing is in the first place. Like entertaining pure thoughts or acting from a place of pure love.

The search for purity is a path and a practice, not a destination. Pure food, like pure roundedness, does not, in reality, exist. It is an ideal. And we are very much meant to enjoy the journey toward it. But woe be our Virgo nature when it makes us lust after purity as an end goal! While the Virgo mind is strong, using it to perfectly define perfection is one of her pitfalls. For instance, highly controlled food intake does not mean that a diet—or the body that receives it—will be pure. In fact, even if you took it to an absolute extreme and ate only air, the air's contaminants would make its ingestion impure. Similarly, spending your entire weekend editing and reediting the same memo does not make every word or comma used perfect.

Throughout Asia sit as many ♍ angry Buddha statues as happy ones. They remind us when enough is enough, to help us extinguish thoughts, emotions, and habits that no longer serve our purpose, in order to purify, grow, and move on.

Purity is an ideal that we strive toward with our nutrition, our work, our state of mind, and anything else we choose. When done with proper Virgo energy, striving can be a process of bettering, perfecting, and purifying yourself that keeps bringing you closer to the authentic you, which is the ultimate source of inner-outer alignment, satisfaction, and fulfillment. And if your Virgo energy can direct that degree of pure personal congruence, well, there's no higher purpose than that.

Virgo vigorously promotes the concept of doing from being, allowing who you are to inspire what you do. For this reason, the constellation's Virgin maiden is typically depicted holding a bundle of wheat. This bundle symbolizes both who she is (a goddess of the earth) and what she does (serve the earth's bounty). With this symbol, the Virgin takes our modern-day notion of the personal-professional division, dissolves the invisible barrier between them, and marries the two.

When this marriage occurs, you have found your purpose. Your purpose is the reason you exist, the unique gift you are here to serve. Some call it a calling. Some are born into it, some develop it, some spend their lives searching for it, and some do not feel that they even have the luxury to look for it. In line with the elusive nature of Plato's forms, many times it is an essence that is better understood in what it is not. For instance, most fast-food employees are pretty sure that temporary shift work is not their true calling. They might not yet know what their calling is, but they know it is not that. That said, even if it is not a calling, everything serves a purpose, even shift work. In the present, perhaps it provides money for rent or food for a family. Or a way to fine-tune the worker's ability to serve by brightening the day of her customers. (Remember: Service is service and no one version is loftier than another. The magic is in the way it occurs.) How will it play into the future? Only hindsight knows for sure. Perhaps it was a stepping-stone to other opportunities, a teacher of important lessons, or in fact, its own career. Whatever *it* is, if you are able to see it for its larger purpose, you are able to feel good and assured about your path.

♍ Virgo Upton Sinclair's book *The Jungle* provoked a national outcry on the state of the food industry in 1906, which resulted in the first federal pure-food statute. A century later the quest continues in the guise of organic, local, and sustainable movements to purify our food today.

Everything you have done, every relationship you have entered, has brought you to where you are now. Your purpose—along with your trajectory to and from it—does not necessarily look a particular way, for it is as unique as you are. It is not necessarily decreed by birth, circumstance, or challenge in achieving it. And even if it is, it might take a lifetime to learn, as it is not necessarily something that even the keen Virgo intellect can figure out. Indeed, it may arise out of trauma, or it may be a soft inner voice or intuition that you need to trust, even if it lies beyond rational thought or conformity with the status quo. It might not look like what you think it should (which is why it can be so darn hard to find). And it might require a total repatterning of your belief systems in order to let go of self-imposed constraints, the type that keeps you playing small as you serve every purpose except your highest one. Virgo, however, is here to encourage you to serve your highest purpose, whatever it is. And that, in turn, is hers. It is how she truly feeds the earth—by feeding your soul.

Lessons

Once upon a time—perhaps when you were a child—you imagined your future. Perhaps you envisioned yourself as a mother, a fairy, a firefighter, or all of the above. Whatever the vision, it was likely powered by a sense of who you were and what you came here to do—a sense that has likely evolved with time. For finding your purpose—let alone living it—is a work in progress. A road on which the things that serve you today might not tomorrow.

When something's or someone's purpose stops serving yours, it is time to give thanks for its service and move on. In this way, Virgo is perpetually removing impurities from your life—inside and out—so that your vision may be brought to life in its purest form. She is always digesting a thought or letting go of a habit—just as her belly assimilates what is necessary for the body and releases what is not. It is a perpetual cleansing of old forms that no longer suffice. She might not know what it all leads to, but she follows a gut sense.

If she ignores this sense, she runs the risk of living an unfulfilling life. She will use superficial perceptions to frame who she is and what she allows in her life. And then nothing will ever stack up or be good enough. Nothing will meet her exacting expectations because she will keep failing to meet her own (those that come from her core). When this occurs, Virgo's inner critic will spiral her into a veritable vortex of judgment of self and others. This vortex might then lead to regular attempts to increase control—typically of health habits and daily routines—as she keeps trying harder and harder to achieve her desired outcome. But if her purpose is misconceived from the beginning, then her trying will be too. And obsession will replace dedication.

Physical manifestations of compulsive Virgo energy may include:

- ★ Rigidly held core
- ★ Militaristic posture
- ★ Shallow or held breath (versus belly breath)
- ★ Other: Poor digestion, disordered eating, indigestion, food allergies, constipation, hernia, ulcers, irritable bowels, hypochondriasis, obsessive behaviors

If the Virgo foregoes control altogether then she forsakes a hallmark of her sign—discipline. Without discipline, her attempts at purification will be irregular or erratic, and she will be a few shades grayer than her truest, purest self. Her service will be commensurately affected and exist in a less pure, less authentic state as well. So whatever is off, her sense of center or her sense of service, this Virgo lesson indicates a sense of self and purpose that still has some ways to go to be fully developed.

Physical manifestations of a permissive Virgo nature may include:

* ★ Weak core
* ★ C-shaped, or lordotic, posture
* ★ Other: Loose or irritable bowels, hernia, binge eating, poor nutrition, indigestion, ulcers, food allergies

How cultivated is your core? Whether it feels compulsive, permissive, or somewhere in between, the key is listening to your body and giving it what it needs. To stretch a tight abdomen or strengthen a weak one, awaken your inner Virgo with the questions and exercises that follow.

Your Body and the Stars

The following will serve as your personal guide to embodying the Virgo stars. Use them to serve with greater purity of purpose.

Questions

* ★ In what ways do you serve your friends? Family? Society? Job?
* ★ Do you feel that you serve purely? If not, what elements in your life would need to come and go in order to feel that way?
* ★ What health routines and rituals do you engage in? What is their purpose? Are they, in fact, serving their purpose?
* ★ Have you found your calling? Whether you have or not, what adjectives would describe it (creative, entrepreneurial, hands-on)? Use your imagination and do not self-censor.
* ★ In what situations do you derive strength from your core? In what situations do you need to?

Exercises

Forearm Plank Plus: To Cultivate Your Core

Do you recall the core exercise on page 90? It is not just a test of core strength but a good core strengthener. It is called plank pose because your body should take the shape of a plank—a board, a long and flat piece of wood. There should be no dipping of the chest nor a rising or dipping of the pelvis . . . but from head to heels, your form should be one straight line. This is easier said than done because it requires

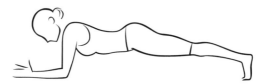

core strength, which is challenging to harness. Given a lifestyle in which we rise from a bed, get into the seat of a car, sit at the computer desk, and lounge on the couch, fitness studios are where we tend to engage our cores. And yet, your core was made for more. You can practice the core strength test as a regular exercise and, to make the pose more challenging, you can add the following movements:

1. Lift your right arm up, parallel to the floor, and hold for fifteen seconds. Return it down.
2. Lift your left arm up, parallel to the floor, and hold for fifteen seconds. Return it down.

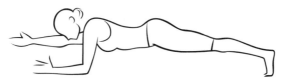

3. Lift the right leg up, parallel to the floor, and hold for fifteen seconds. Return it down.

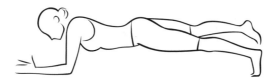

4. Lift the left leg up, parallel to the floor, and hold for fifteen seconds. Return it down.

5. Lift your left leg *and* right arm up, parallel to the floor. Hold for fifteen seconds. Return them to the ground.

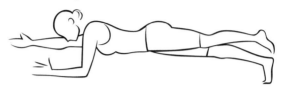

6. Lift your right leg *and* left arm up, parallel to the floor. Hold for fifteen seconds. Return them to the ground.

7. Gently lower yourself to the ground; relax for a moment before getting up.

To decrease the intensity of the pose, drop your knees to the floor and enter into a tabletop position, from which you may raise your arms and legs as instructed above.

Either way, use this exercise as a way of locating your core, engaging it, and allowing the rest of you to move from it. In time, this routine awareness of your core will help you harness its principles of stabilization, center of mass, and balance in all of your activities. In other words: take your core out of the gym and engage it throughout the rest of your sitting, standing, and walking day.

Supine Star Stretch: To Radiate from Your Core

Every star has a core, including Spica, the brightest star of the Virgo constellation. The core is the source of a star's energy. It is here that proton particles collide with enough speed that they stick to each other and create a huge amount of energy through nuclear fusion. This energy both fuels the core and radiates outward into the radiation zone—the next layer of the star—for further use. Your body may be likened to a five-pointed star; your core generates the musculoskeletal fuel that powers *your* radiation zones—head and neck, upper and lower limbs—allowing them to energize in their own right and transmit that energy even further (like helping your arms lift a heavy object). Use this exercise to practice being the star you are and radiate energy outward from your core:

Spica looks like one star, but it is at least two, each larger and hotter than our sun. And based on observations of its light, some astronomers even think that Spica is not composed of two stars . . . but five!

1. Lie on your back on the floor. Turn your body into a five-pointed star by extending your arms outward along the floor, making a V shape around your head, and spreading your legs.

2. Relax in this position and feel how your body's energy is comfortably dispersed.

3. Now fold your arms, legs, and head in toward your chest so that you become a tight human ball, contracting every muscle in this position.

4. With purpose, extend your head and limbs outward, back into the star formation on the floor. All five points—two hands and two feet plus one head—should reach the floor at exactly the same time. Do not let them drop carelessly, forcefully, or one-by-one to the ground. Know where they are going and put power and purpose behind placing them there. When all of you reaches the floor, your star position should be active and engaged, all the way through your fingers and toes. Release excess tension from the head, neck, and shoulders.

5. Come back into a ball and then re-extend. Repeat this ten times. Breathe.

Did you notice that your ability to place your head and limbs with precision is directly related to the physical engagement of your core? The more you concentrate on your center as the source of your limbs' strength, the more powerful and purposeful their movements will be.

Mountain Pose: To Return to Center

On a mountain stands an oak tree and a reed. One day, in the midst of a storm, the sturdy oak breaks at the trunk while the supple reed, still standing, merely bends. It sways in the gusty winds and, after the storm ends, returns to its upright position. Be the reed, standing strong in your purpose but supple enough to weather life's inevitable storms. Mountain pose will help you connect to your center . . . so that you can throw yourself from it, only to return to it again. Ultimately, no one can distract you from your center but you.

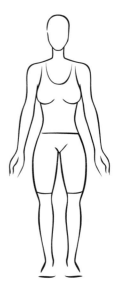

1. Stand with your feet hip distance apart, in their natural parallel position. Form a firm foundation by lifting and spreading out your toes to place them evenly on the floor. Center your weight between both feet.

2. Engage your inner arches, and feel that engagement rise through your legs and thighs. Very slightly turn your thighs inward.

3. Lower your tailbone toward the floor while lifting your navel.

4. Engage your core so that it becomes a center of strength.

5. Gently open your chest and shoulders; feel your shoulder blades firm and broad against your back. Your forearms hang by your sides, with your palms engaged and facing front, fingers lengthened and alive.

6. Stack your neck on top of your torso (not in front), with your head resting in neutral, chin parallel to the floor. Release any neck and shoulder tension. Soften your gaze and breathe.

7. When you feel strong and centered in this pose, close your eyes. Notice the natural swaying that occurs.

8. Now, increase the sway to the right side until you almost fall—but don't. Return yourself to your centered position with as minimal movement and effort as possible.

9. Now tip your weight to the left side, followed by a return to center. Do the same toward the front and back. Play around with how far you can go without falling, returning yourself to center after each time.

10. When you are done rediscovering center, return to mountain pose and hold it for thirty seconds before exiting.

Take your yoga off the mat: just as you try to re-create the centered sensation of mountain pose in all yoga poses, try to re-create it throughout the rest of your life as well—in body, mind, and spirit.

Breath of Fire: To Purify

Within the yoga system, the physical body is believed to connect to subtle energy bodies (mental body, emotional body) through the *chakras*. In Sanskrit, these "spinning wheels," unite your manifold natures. There are seven major chakras arranged vertically in the body along a channel that runs through your midline; each corresponds to a particular region of the body. The third chakra, for example, corresponds to the abdomen and its contents. Apart from regulating the physical region, it is also believed to govern your sense of self—not only your core identity (pun intended) but also the power, confidence, and vitality with which you project this internal sense to the outside world. The fire within, so to speak. And not just the digestive one!

The fire that fuels who you are and what you are here to do every day. Use the following breath to revitalize your inner fire, burning any impurities, such as outdated thoughts or emotions, that stand in its—and your—way.

1. Find a comfortable seat on the floor, sitting cross-legged upon a cushion, pillow, or block if needed (if cross-legged is not possible, find an easeful position sitting upright on a floor; if this position is not possible, sit on a chair). Rest your palms on your knees. Your spine is long, and your chin is subtly tucked in toward your chest. Close your eyes.
2. Take a deep inhale though the nose and allow your chest and belly to fully expand with the breath.
3. Exhale through the nose, pushing out the air completely (as you would from a balloon).
4. Now, begin to breathe more vigorously with equal emphasis on the inhalation and exhalation. Start slowly and establish a steady rhythm. Increase to a quick but comfortable pace (it will feel like fast sniffing). Keep the chest and stomach relaxed. Allow them to pulse on their own with each breath.
5. Continue for one minute.

In yogic tradition, Breath of Fire is believed to clean both the body and the mind. It is recommended that you wait at least two hours after eating to perform this breath to allow your digestive system to be as clean and pure as possible. If you feel uncomfortable or lightheaded while doing it, please stop. You can resume it later and less intensely.

Mindful Eating: To Be Purposeful
Everything has a purpose. But if you are stuck in your own perspective, you might miss it. A great example is food, which is not only a full sensory experience but is also fuel for your cells. These days, though, who knows what purpose food serves? Perhaps it serves your mind, as you decide the XYZ diet makes intellectual sense for certain reasons. Perhaps the food provides comfort for your emotions. Perhaps it serves the demands of your day as you consume it while walking down the sidewalk or while reading the computer screen at your desk. Practice being purposeful by being purposeful with your food. A close connection to food—given her connection to both Earth and the belly—is a Virgo birthright. And given that the mental master

Mercury is her ruling planet, so is her mind. Mindful eating, then, becomes a great way for the Virgo to practice a purposeful life.

1. Choose a time when you are alone (no people, no reading, no electronics, no distractions).
2. Choose a bite-sized piece of food to enjoy (like a dried apricot, chocolate, a nut).
3. Before you place the food in your mouth, spend one minute otherwise consuming it: Rotate it with your fingers and feel its texture and see it from all sides. Smell it. If there was wrapping, what sound did it make as you removed it?
4. Place the goody in your mouth. *Before* chewing, roll your tongue over it and roll it around in your mouth so that it touches your palate and the inner cheeks. Close your eyes to heighten the sensation.
5. Begin chewing—fully and completely. How long can you chew before swallowing?

Virgo pitfalls include judgment, control, and self-criticism, all stemming from that strong mind. So, as part of this practice, leave those traits at home. They have no place at this meal—just enjoy and explore!

Offering: To Serve

Ancient Hindu texts mention a Sanskrit word, *prasad*, that refers to an offering, a gracious gift. In the earliest writings, this gift was a state of being—a state of grace possessed by gods, goddesses, and sages. Later, the offerings became more material, a ritual offering in which food, for example, was devoted to a deity for blessing and then distributed to followers—as a blessing—on the deity's behalf. This grace—whether in conceptual or physical form—is how Virgo serves. Practice this form of service with your own offering:

1. Choose a corner of your community that you would like to bless or otherwise wish goodwill; it might be friends, family, colleagues, or neighbors.
2. Choose the blessing you would like to bestow (forgiveness, love, joy, gratitude, abundance).
3. Choose the form(s) in which you would like to offer the gift (it might be fruit, flower, dessert, coin, or craft).

4. Create a space in which you can bless the gift in a meaningful way (like the corner of the bedroom or living room). Traditional *prasad* involves the placement of the object upon an altar with candles and religious statues. That said, creating a sacred space for yourself by holding the object and placing your positive intentions upon it is enough. Whatever gives it meaning to and through you.

5. Give your *prasad!* With love, joy, and no expectation of anything—even a smile—in return. Your service is fulfilled.

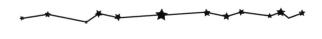

Summary

★ Your abdomen is the region related to Virgo. Its visceral contents allow food to provide a nutritional service for you, just as its core muscles provide a stabilizing one.

★ Virgo is the sixth sign of the zodiac cycle. Its energy pertains to serving a purpose that allows all other people, places, and things to serve theirs.

★ If your purity-seeking Virgo nature gets too compulsive or, conversely, too permissive, your abdomen might experience different symptoms (e.g., weak core, poor digestion).

★ Center your inner Virgo through questions, exercises, and meditations that focus on your abdomen. Use them to get in touch with your life's calling, remembering that it is a continual journey, not a finite outcome.

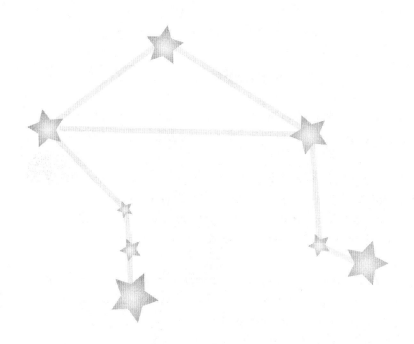

8

Back of the Scales

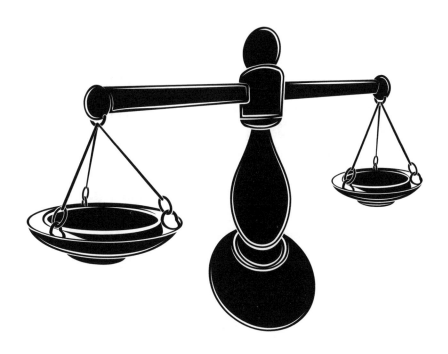

♎ LIBRA

Birth date: September 23–October 22
Body region: Lower Back
Theme: Balance Your Scales of
Truth with Grace

Libra launches the second half of the zodiac cycle. Recall that the first half—Aries through Virgo—constructed the self. Now you enter Libra, with the needed foundation to dive deep into the other, and to do so without losing yourself in the midst, because your self-development is definitely not done, just continuing in a new direction. One that asks you—with all your personal hopes, dreams, and desires—to meaningfully accommodate others. It is a fine line to walk as you question where you end and others begin. It requires balancing multiple scales of truth, a task that the sign of Libra is here to graciously do.

Your Body: Lower Back

The back is the region of your body that spans from the pelvic brim to the base of your neck. While the same spine (vertebral column) and most of the muscles run throughout its broad expanse, the back is commonly considered to consist of two subregions: upper and lower. The upper back is discussed with Leo in chapter 6: "Heart of the Lion," as the region that relates to the thoracic spine. The lower back is farther down, relates to the lumbar spine, and is the region associated with Libra.

The lumbar region is distinctive for its large vertebral bones. Their size is required to support all of the weight above it—from your head, neck, arms, and back—while balancing the movements of your torso. To do so, your back has its own support mechanisms in place, like intervertebral discs between adjacent vertebrae for shock absorption and a system of ligaments for stability. There are also deep muscles that help the bones, disks, and ligaments stay in place, like the erector spinae and transversospinalis groups. These deep stabilizers support the back's entire structure and function; they are the ones that dynamically keep your back "straight" when you're sitting on a stool (i.e., with no built-in back support).

 To the eye, your back looks straight. But the vertebral column is actually shaped like an *S*, which is what creates the curves of the upper and lower back in addition to that of the sacrum and neck. These curves help support the torso against gravity.

They are also the muscles believed to be involved in lower back pain, which is a common reason for visits to primary care offices nationwide. Lower back pain may stem from many sources including overusing the back, misusing it, or a combination of the two (as in frequently lifting heavy objects with improper posture). Your lumbar spine is stable, but it is also mobile, and increased mobility results in increased injury susceptibility. Especially if you are not giving your back what it needs to properly function.

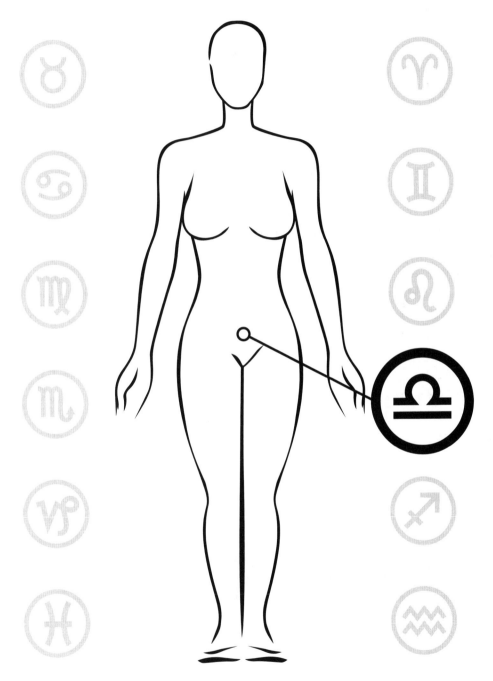

See appendix C for the skeletal structure of the lower back.

In other words, your back has "got your back." But do you give it the support it needs to support you? If its muscles and joints are weak and unstable, or poorly supported by the abdomen, they will not be able to balance everything that comes on top.

And balance is the name of Libra's game! If you cannot balance your own weight, how are you supposed to effectively do the same for others? Knowing how to balance others begins by knowing how to balance you. After all, when your inner Libra is balancing the weight of the world, you want it to come from a stable place. If it does not, then you might lift a box one day and—bam!—throw out your back. Even though it seems as if this accident happened all of a sudden, chances are it was a long time in the making. The structures around your lumbar spine were shifting out of their natural balance slowly but surely for some time; whatever you lifted happened to be the final straw that broke the camel's back.

There is no need to wait for an injury, however, to give your back (or any part of your body) what it needs. Every physical structure—from your body to your abode—requires a backbone for support, and your back is no exception. In fact, it is your foundation. How well does yours support you? To see, try cobra pose:

1. Lie flat on your belly. Hands are flat on the floor, directly under your shoulders; fingers are engaged and elbows hugged in toward your sides. Legs are elongated, with the tops of your feet pressed into the floor.
2. Inhale and begin to extend your elbows, lifting your chest off the floor. The lift should arise from the strength of your lower back, not your arms. Hips and legs stay on the ground; buttocks are engaged but not gripped. Be mindful not to hold your breath!
3. Extend your arms only to the height at which you can maintain a connection between the front of your pelvis and the floor—which might mean that your elbows remain bent. Make sure that your head and neck are aligned as a continuation of the rest of your spine and not overly extended or flexed; your gaze should fall diagonally on the floor in front of you.
4. Depress your shoulders, firm your shoulder blades against your back, and lift your hands two inches off of the floor. Notice if the height of your back lowers as a result.
5. Wherever you are in space, hold the pose for thirty seconds, breathing.
6. Release to the floor on an exhalation.

The height of your back when your hands are off the floor (and your buttocks are relaxed) represents the strength intrinsic to your back and, specifically, its extensor muscles. You should be able to maintain one height comfortably for thirty seconds. The stronger your back becomes, the higher it will be able to lift off the floor. Of course, strength needs to be balanced with stretch so your back does not become too tight or rigid. Instead, it should possess a flexible stability that allows it to give and receive support both internally and externally. Which, perhaps, comes from yet another Libra-esque balance between saying no to others and yes to you.

The Stars: Libra

Balance Your Scales of Truth with Grace

Imagine balancing on one foot. Even though you might think you are balanced, is your standing foot truly still? No. Its many muscles, along with those of the ankle, are making myriad micro-adjustments. These adjustments act on the joints, helping to keep you erect by everting your foot if it is too inverted and flexing if it is too extended. All in all, while you do not appear to be moving, your balance is a dynamic movement, a dance between your foot and the floor.

> This fine-tuning also occurs internally, as many substances—like iodine—are required for your body's maintenance but only in certain doses. You need just enough iodine to maintain your thyroid functions—too much may result in toxicity and too little in hypothyroidism.

The key to establishing your inner balance is therefore predicated upon the knowledge that balance is not a finite or static point in time or space. That it exists *within* any given spectrum and is manifest through the choices you continue to make (those micro-adjustments), in proportions that work for you. And you can access this balance by invoking your Libra sensibility.

While Libra's constellation—the Scales—is in the sky, the sign provides an earthly reminder that there are invisible scales hanging all around us. From work demands and self-care, to portions of vegetables versus dessert, equilibrating the sides of these scales requires you to engage your inner Libra—to be aware of which side needs more weight, more focus, more time, and more attention. This perpetual calibrating is what keeps you feeling like you are getting what you need *while* attending to others. Sure, maybe you could do with a little bit more or a little less but, overall, you feel balanced, in check, supported—like you are getting what you need while responding fairly to the environment and people around you.

Everyone's inner Libra is called to balance his scales. Heck, even our government has a system of checks and balances, a way to ensure that no one branch of government exerts too much force on the nation. (Not surprisingly, it was a Libra—the former chief justice of the supreme court John Marshall—who helped balance the country's governing equation by giving the judicial branch parity with the other two.) Sure, sometimes the pendulum will swing to one of the branches, but it will not be there for long. The nature of a pendulum is to swing between the ends of a spectrum and pass its equilibrium in between, and the same is true for you. While, for the pendulum, the force that equilibrates it is gravity, you have your inner Libra to guide you toward a fluctuating harmony that works for you. An inner ability that not only helps you find and maintain balance but also do so in a manner aligned with your inner truth.

> Libra engages in its own heavenly balancing act as the zodiac sign that marks the autumnal equinox, a time when day and night are of roughly equal length.

The Libra civil rights activist Mahatma Gandhi invoked truth in his movement for Indian independence. In fact, he coined the term *satyagraha* (*satya* implying truth and love, *graha* implying firmness and force) to describe his tenet—a determined but nonviolent resistance to British imperialism. As Gandhi explained, "This Truth is not merely the Truth we are expected to speak, it is that which alone is, which constitutes the stuff of which all things are made, which subsists by virtue of its own power, which is not supported by anything else but supports everything that exists. Truth alone is eternal, everything else is momentary. . . it is not a blind law. It governs the entire universe."[1]

> After his followers conducted acts of violence, Gandhi realized that his teachings of *Satyagraha* required greater training in order to be exemplified in word and deed. He subsequently suspended the campaign, although it was ultimately considered successful.

When accessing a greater truth, however, it must be brought to the individual level in order to be lived as your personal truth; otherwise, it cannot effect change. And that can get tricky. Because even if there is one overarching truth, it is understood in as many ways as it has seekers—even within just you. For each side of a story presents its own version of the truth, and Libra sees them all. This part of you knows that not one side or the other alone is valid but that all can be valid simultaneously, and to the greatest extent possible, they should all be respected. The challenge, however, is not to negate your own truth when surrounded by others'. Sure, your inner Libra happens to be a natural people-pleaser but, at the end of the day, your truth describes the fullest and most authentic expression of you.

So the key is to be in touch with and maintain your own true Libra, even when it conflicts with others. Thus enters grace.

Consider John Godfrey Saxe's version of the Indian legend "The Blind Men and the Elephant": Six men, feeling different parts of the same elephant, each comes up with a different interpretation of what the elephant is—a wall, a spear, a snake, a tree, a fan, and a rope. Though "each was partly in the right . . . all were in the wrong!" ♎

You have probably heard the phrase "by the grace of God" many times, but what does it really mean? Well, *grace* in the New Testament is translated from the Greek *charis*, which refers to a favor that God gives freely; for instance, salvation to sinners and blessings for the unrepentant.

While in the New Testament it is a religious term, grace is a universal concept. Everyone is able to bestow blessings, every day and in a variety of forms. Like the gracious host who readily accommodates his guests' culinary preferences, the gracious loser who sincerely shakes his opponent's hand, or the graceful ballerina whose performance for her audience belies bloodied feet. Grace, then, is not only the act but also a quality with which the act is performed.

The difference between acting graciously and people-pleasing is that in the former, you are well aware of your truth and *choose* not to give it a voice for what you perceive to be the greater good. Truth is in its knowing, and the ego's desire to blurt it out does not make it any more or less true. In fact, many times silence maintains truth better than words. In the latter, people-pleasing, you might not be aware of your truth or you might be; either way, you are going against it for some ulterior motive like winning affection, attaining approval, or otherwise using it as a means to some intentional or unintentional end. The result ultimately speaks for itself, not as the heavenly satisfaction that grace implies, but as underlying resentment and overall drain.

If our Libras were to lead the way and we were to truly live with grace, our world would witness a time of greater peace, harmony, and stability. In a way, it would resemble the Golden Age, the highest of the Greek Ages of Man. According to the ancient Greek poet Hesiod, this era was one of harmony, prosperity, and a race of beings who were the golden children of gods. Astraea, the star maiden, presided over the age until time passed and humankind deteriorated, becoming self-centered, greedy, and violent. The descent continued and, after the Golden Age tumbled into Silver and then Bronze (our current age is Iron), she left. She could not stand the lack of grace, and her gift of it was totally lost on this new world. So she returned to the heavens, where she currently holds Libra's Scales and supports humankind's endeavors from above. A

While Astraea holds Libra's Scales, she does so while standing in the constellation of Virgo. In this capacity, she is also considered one of the celestial maidens of Virgo, along with Isis, Demeter, and the Virgin Mary. She is also associated with Dike, goddess of justice.

sad end to the tale? Your inner Libra would say, "Maybe and maybe not." For even though we lost the guidance of the goddess here on Earth, we are now tasked to access the same attributes within ourselves. And this self-seeking and -reliance may be a far richer means of attaining well-being than having someone do it in our stead.

Lessons

Inside and out, Libra is here to balance the world's many truths, and in a gracious way. Grace comes naturally to this sign's energy, which intrinsically values congeniality and harmony. Your Libra, then, makes for a wonderful diplomat who can maintain the peace or a lawyer who can argue each side of every coin. In turn, readily attuning to the world's needs makes the Libra likeable to all.

Libra's fundamental focus is on partnerships and relationships, on the *you* or *us* versus the *me*. And the lesson with this energy is to make sure that your Libra does not lose his integrity in attuning to everyone else's needs. Covering up his own truth—or not standing up for it—can many times make it easier to keep the peace. No one likes ruffled feathers less than the Libra. But by not rocking the boat, he inadvertently chooses superficiality to command his word and deed. He will then rise in corporate ranks not because he is living an inner truth but because he is catering to appearances and expectations. In the process, he might even tell (white) lies about his opinions, never say no, and smile with the veneer of false grace—all in the effort to make others happy.

Libras easily blend into the crowd. This is true for the constellation as well: none of its stars are of first magnitude, making it relatively faint. Two of its stars actually used to belong to the constellation Scorpio, forming its claws.

But that can only last so long. People-pleasing is tiring, especially when the Libra side of you pleases everyone except yourself. It is not uncommon, then, for your Libra to reach a point where he feels spent, fatigued, and generally out of balance. Physical problems might even arise to help him rebalance his equation, effectively forcing him to attend to the rest and self-support that he needs. In other words, the Libra needs to rediscover his own backbone. Lower back pain typically occurs when the back muscles are too weak or too tight (which is not the same thing as strong) and typically in the context of poor abdominal support (see chapter 8: "Belly of the Virgin").

DAVID FURLONG

ILLUMINATING
THE
SHADOW

TRANSMUTING THE DARK SIDE OF THE PSYCHE

ISBN 978-0-9559795-6-9

ILLUMINATING THE SHADOW:
Transmuting the Dark Side of the Psyche
by David Furlong

David Furlong's latest book, *Illuminating the Shadow*, is a wonderful, erudite account of the human psyche, particularly in its wounded and hidden aspects. First we are introduced to the concept of the Shadow in films, literature, myth, metaphor and Fairy Tales, before learning how it manifests at a personal, public and collective level. Finally, we are taught how to learn from and integrate this aspect of ourselves, and of the human condition. *Illuminating the Shadow* is full of practical insights drawn from Furlong's work as a therapist, with exercises to help the reader explore and make peace with him or herself. It is the sort of book that deserves more than one reading; that asks to be borrowed and lent so that the wisdom contained within can be shared as widely as possible.

Dr Fiona Bowie, King's College London & the Afterlife Research Centre Author of the bestselling *Anthropology of Religion* (Blackwell)

Illuminating the Shadow explores a rich breadth of academic knowledge and everyday life experience with great depth and wisdom. Scholarly exposition of shadow through history, the arts and sciences provides far-reaching insights for human nature and global society. Story, myth and metaphor show how we express and try to understand our own complexity, divine mystery and the struggle between good and evil at personal and collective levels. And bringing dark psyche into the light shows shadow in relief, not to be eliminated but illuminated since, in its vital integrative function, it is both teacher and healer. Therapeutic examples and exercises in shadow work demonstrate the journey into light and compassionate love, with free will continuously informed by evolving consciousness, that points us towards full relationship with the living human God, and with our selves and each other. For the advancement of mental and spiritual health, this eminently practical book deserves a wide readership.

Dr David McDonald, Consultant Psychiatrist and Advisor in the Church of England's Healing Ministry

---

Published by Atlanta Books in association with Troubador Publishing. Order your *signed* copy today at the discount price of £12.98 incl. p&p. Available from David Furlong, Myrtles Como Road, Malvern, Worcs., WR14 2TH.   Email: atlanta@dial.pipex.com or online from **www.davidfurlong.co.uk/books_shadow.htm**

If the deep back muscles are tight, the Libra might be holding on to support structures for dear life. Perhaps his routines for self-support are too rigid, too limited. Or based upon truths so tightly held they have become dogma. In other words, they are *too* supportive in that they are limiting him to one place when what he requires is a greater range.

Physical manifestations of a resisting Libra nature may include:

★ Tight, tense lower back muscles
★ Muscle spasms
★ Limited range of motion
★ Flat back posture
★ Acute pain with sudden movements
★ Other: Kidney or adrenal imbalance (In accordance with Libra's balancing act, these organs, which are deep to the lower back, come in pairs.)

If the scales are tipped the other way, the deep back muscles cannot support either themselves or the surrounding structures, which makes the entire region more susceptible to injury. It is as if—at the physical level—no one's got your back. Or perhaps you have support systems in place but they are all external (like friends) versus internal (like self-confidence), which makes you likely to crumble if they were to ever disappear. In either case, the back can no longer support the weight of the current lifestyle that your Libra energy is leading.

Physical manifestations of a yielding Libra nature may include:

★ Sore, strained back muscles
★ Pain or weakness with physical expenditure (e.g., lifting)
★ C-shaped or lordotic posture
★ Pain and symptoms consistent with joint degeneration
★ Other: Kidney or adrenal imbalance

How supportive is your back? Whether it feels resisting, yielding, or somewhere in between, the key is listening to your body and giving it what it needs. To stretch a tight lower back or strengthen a weak one, awaken your inner Libra with the questions and exercises that follow.

Your Body and the Stars

The following will serve as your personal guide to embodying the story of the Libra stars. Use them to balance your scales of truth with grace.

Questions

★ Do you feel that your life is balanced? What area(s) of your life may be out of balance? How can you rebalance the scales in your life?

★ What truths do you hold that are fundamental to who you are and what you do? Which one is at the top of the list? How do you incorporate it in your daily life?

★ Do you know where you end and others begin?

★ Would you say that you exhibit the quality of grace in your daily life? How? When? During what situations do you wish you could invoke more grace?

★ Does your back support you in your current lifestyle and endeavors? What needs to happen for you and your back to feel even better supported?

Exercises

Half-Boat Pose: For Balance, Strength, and Support

Have you ever seen a picture of a cobra with its head raised several inches off the floor? Thanks to its muscular makeup, this snake can elevate about one-third of its body as the rest remains on the ground. It is a balancing act that is true for you as well, and one that you practiced earlier in the chapter with cobra pose (which you can keep practicing). It employed your back extensors and stabilizers to enable and maintain the lift. With boat pose, you balance the back's strength with that of the abdomen for further core support.

1. Sit upright with knees bent and feet flat on the floor. Arms are by your sides with the palms planted next to your hips.
2. Engage your core and—keeping your torso straight—raise one leg and then the other so that both shins come parallel to the floor. Press your palms firmly into the floor to help you until you are balanced on your sitting bones.

3. Once you have found your balance, raise your arms alongside your legs so your arms are parallel to each other and the floor. Hands are engaged, fingers together, with palms facing in toward the legs. Make sure to keep your shoulder blades flat on your back so that you do not hunch forward. Tilt the head slightly toward the chest to maintain an elongated neck.

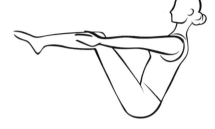

4. Remain, breathing, in the pose for thirty seconds without dropping your legs; work your way toward one minute. Your abdominal wall should be engaged but not tense.

5. To release, lower your feet to the floor and rock up to a sitting position, aided by your hands, and then slowly lower yourself so that you are flat on your back and can stretch yourself out on the floor.

If boat pose offers too much core work for now, keep your hands at your sides, supporting you on the floor. On the other hand, if you want more of a workout or to enter into the full expression of the pose, straighten your legs while maintaining a neutral torso. But remember that spinal support is most important, so never sacrifice leg height for the integrity of your spine!

Rolling Like a Ball: To Move toward Balance

Around the turn of the seventeenth century, the multi-talented astronomer-mathematician-scientist-philosopher Galileo Galilei discovered the key characteristics of a pendulum by observing chandeliers swinging in a cathedral. Each chandelier was moving back and forth through its equilibrium point, displaced by currents of air. The human body can, likewise, be seen as a pendulum; your lower limb (from hip to foot), for instance, acts as a physical pendulum when it swings forward to take a step.

This exercise allows your entire body to replicate this arc as you roll from one end (sitting bones) to the other (shoulders). As you roll, allow your back to relax in order to gracefully move between ends, noticing that most of your time in this exercise is actually spent in between.

1. Sit upright on your sitting bones on a padded surface, such as a mat. Draw your knees toward your chest and clasp your hands over your shins.

2. Form a C curve with your spine as you drop your shoulders, widen your back, and deepen your abdomen. Your neck should maintain the natural elongation of the spine.

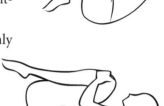

3. Lift your feet off of the ground to balance on your sitting bones.
4. Exhale to deepen the C curve and roll back. Roll only to the level of the shoulders, being careful not to roll onto the neck.
5. Maintaining the C curve, inhale to roll forward and onto your sitting bones.
6. Repeat five to ten times.

Feel crooked or off balance? Keep practicing and focus on your spine as the centerline.

Standing Spinal Twists: To See Many Truths

The body is a finely calibrated machine that uses sensory input from your environment—many times without your even realizing it—to make decisions about how to keep you balanced. That is why, for instance, you can take a misstep off of a curb that is only three inches high, and yet it feels like a much bigger drop and you land with a thud. Sensory input was missing. Your head is the primary commander of this input, especially the inner ear, and your neck is the region that moves the head (see chapter 2: "Head of the Ram" and chapter 3: "Neck of Bull," respectively). But your lower back is what supports them both and, by virtue of its own movements, allows them to take in an even wider scope by rotating right and left. By enjoying a greater rotation around your body's central axis, you are then able to appreciate the world's fuller extent. You can better see the different parts to the world and how each has a different story to tell, a different truth to hold. And the more you are aware of them, the more you will be able to integrate them internally and accommodate them externally.

1. Stand with your feet hip distance apart with a slight bend in your knees. Allow your arms to hang loosely by your sides.
2. Rotate your torso to the right, allowing your arms to swing so that the left moves in front of the body and the right moves in back. Rotate to the left, with

the right hand swinging in front of the body and the left behind. Allow the twist to arise from the lower back; your pelvis should remain facing square in front of you.

3. Continue the alternating rotations, allowing your body to swing freely between the two, as if you were a Maypole.

4. Swing for a total of twenty rotations.

Now be aware without seeing: close your eyes and continue the twists. Believe it or not, closing your eyes will maximize the range of motion and fluidity of the rotations. Instead of supporting yourself with your gaze, support your back's rotations with a neutral pelvis and firmly planted feet.

Satnam Meditation: For Awareness of Truth

In the simplest of terms, *sat* translates from Gurmukhi to "truth" and *nam* to "name." So saying *satnam* is a way of acknowledging your true nature—your divinity. It is like saying, "I recognize my true self." Ancient yogis believe that this meditation is a first step to manifesting the essential truth on our material plane.

1. Find a comfortable seat on the floor, sitting cross-legged upon a cushion, pillow, or block if needed (if cross-legged is not possible, find an easeful position sitting upright on a floor; if this position is not possible, sit on a chair).

2. In its fullest expression, *satnam* is a four-syllable word pronounced *sa-ta-na-ma*. *Sa* relates to totality, *ta* life, *na* death, and *ma* resurrection.[2] As you pronounce each syllable throughout the entire meditation, you will touch each thumb to each fingertip (using both hands). On the sound of *sa*, touch the thumb to the index finger, *ta* to the middle finger, *na* to the ring, and *ma* to the pinkie. Then start again with *sa*.

3. Chant the mantra (repeated sounds) out loud for one minute.

4. Whisper it for one minute.

5. Internally repeat it for five minutes.

6. Whisper it for one minute.

7. Chant it out loud for one minute.

8. Sit quietly for a moment before arising.

While *satnam* is especially popular within Kundalini yoga, its doppelgänger—*namaste*—is more frequently heard in other forms. It is typically used for closure at the end of a class to impart a sense of respect and honor, as in, "The divine light within me bows to the divine light within you."

The total time is nine minutes, but work your way up toward a full fifteen minutes—five minutes for chanting and whispering plus ten minutes for internal repetition. And don't forget the thumb mudras (gestures) to go with your mantra.

Alternate Nostril Breath: To Balance Yourself and Others

Have you ever heard anyone say, "Just take a deep breath and count to ten" when you were angry, or do you have a friend always reminding you to exhale when you're visibly stressed? Whether they realize it or not, this is sage advice because a slow, deep breath invokes the parasympathetic division of your nervous system, the rest-and-digest response that allows you to calm and center. This breath also centers you metaphysically, by balancing both sides of your energetic body. The left, or yin, side is the part of you that represents intuition, reception, and relations; the right side is the dynamic yang, the fire that is you as actor, creator, and doer. Both parts live within you. But chances are that, if you live in Western society, you have more greatly cultivated your yang. Bring all of you back into balance by cultivating the yin *with* the yang. This will help you maintain the energy and grace necessary to keep doing for others and yourself.

1. Find a comfortable cross-legged seat on the floor. Turn your phone off and set an alarm for five minutes.
2. Your left hand rests in your lap with the palm up while your right hand forms the *vishnu* mudra: index and middle fingers flexed in toward the palm while the thumb, ring, and pinkie fingers remain extended.
3. Close your eyes and take a couple of deep breaths in and out through the nose.
4. Following an exhale, gently close your right nostril with your right thumb. Taking care to modulate your breathing evenly, inhale through your left nostril for a slow count of four.
5. Then close your left nostril with your right ring finger and open up your right nostril. Exhale slowly for four counts.
6. Inhale for four counts through your right nostril.
7. Close your right nostril with your right thumb and open your left nostril. Exhale slowly for four counts.
8. Begin the cycle again and repeat for five minutes.
9. When finished, release the hand mudra and return to normal breathing for a few moments before getting up.

This technique can be done for any amount of time, and even just one minute of concentrated breath helps equilibrate your right and left sides. So whether you want a morning practice to harmonize body and mind, or are stressed at work, or are in the midst of a family gathering, all you need is one minute of personal time to help you reestablish balance in your life.

Any of the Above: To Cultivate Grace

Grace is a quality, an essence. It lives throughout your body and its movements, your perceptions and words, your feelings and behaviors. It is typically characterized as flowing, fluid, and elegant. An internal beauty that infuses its surroundings with calm.

Anything can be done with grace, because for any *what*, grace is the *how*. So how can you walk gracefully, talk gracefully, and otherwise be a graceful human being? With awareness—awareness as to what quality (and there are many to choose from) infuses your daily patterns *and* how these patterns both intentionally and unintentionally affect others. Because grace is a practice of awareness, practice makes perfect. Pick one of the above exercises that you already did and do it again, with grace. Repeat as many times as necessary to feel graceful while maintaining the integrity of the movement.

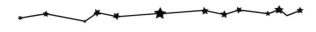

Summary

- ★ Your lower back is the region related to Libra. With the largest vertebrae of the spine, it supports you so you can support others too.
- ★ Libra is the seventh sign of the zodiac cycle. Its energy pertains to balance. Whether it's your truth, his truth, or society's, Libra gracefully honors the authenticity of all.
- ★ If your people-pleasing Libra nature tips the scales toward either too limited or too yielding, your lower back might experience different symptoms (e.g., muscle soreness, ache, strain.)
- ★ Balance your inner Libra through questions, exercises, and activities that focus on your lower back. Use them to tune in to—and re-equilibrate—your body-mind-spirit needs, just as you do for others.

Notes

1. Yogesh Chadha, *Gandhi: A Life* (New York: John Wiley & Sons, 1997), 113.

2. Georg Feuerstein, *The Yoga Tradition: Its History, Literature, Philosophy and Practice* (Prescott, AZ: Hohm Press, 1998), 448.

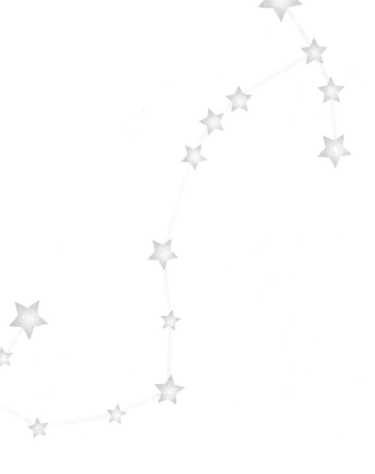

9

Sacrum of the Scorpio

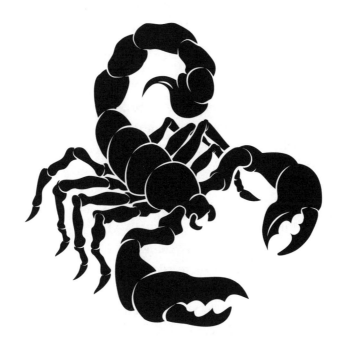

♏ SCORPIO

Birth date: October 23–November 21
Body region: Sacral Center
Theme: Die, Transform, and Soar

S corpio occupies a special place in the zodiac, demarcating a change in tempo between the signs that come before and after it. In other words, it is now time to move beyond your daily state of affairs to your connection with the larger fabric of life. In order for this to take place, however, you need to metaphorically die in order to be reborn. Enter Scorpio. This sign comes straight from the underworld to uproot the subconscious patterns that you have carried through lifetimes. It is a burning of karma that sheds layers of skin, time and time again. This eternal cathar-sis is the essence of Scorpio, who is ready to take the plunge and risk losing it all for the sake of regeneration. Each death brings this transformation as Scorpio's Phoenix crashes and burns, only to rise from the ashes and soar once again.

Your Body: Sacrum

The sacrum is a collection of five fused bones at the end of your spine. The triangular bone comes below your lower back (lumbar spine) and above your tailbone (coccyx). The Latin root for the bone is *os sacrum* and means "sacred," called so because of an ancient belief that the soul resides there (perhaps even relating to where babies' souls are cradled while in utero).

The sacrum forms a greater region—a big, bony basin—along with your pelvis. Each half of the pelvis forms the front and sides of this basin, and the sacrum unites the two halves at the back. They come together at the sacroiliac joints, named for the connection between the sacrum and each of the ilia, which are the winged pelvic bones; these joints are mobile enough to shift your pelvis as you walk but do not have nearly the range of the synovial joints of the rest of your back. In fact, their move-ments—while important—are fairly minimal because of the joints' need to impart stability. After all, these two small joints are the only place in the body where your entire torso connects to your lower limbs!

Additionally, stability is necessary because your sacral region, or center, encom-passes the area traditionally known as the womb. So, apart from it being the nidus of birth in a metaphysical sense, it is very much so physically as well. Its contents include female sexual organs like the uterus and ovaries, all necessary for having a child, as well as male reproductive anatomy, like the prostate gland. Plus, the features of the pelvis itself help develop and birth a child, which is why a woman's pelvis has wider angles and larger inlets and outlets than a man's. With these distinctive features, the pelvis is one of the few bones in the body by which we can distinguish the gender of a skeleton.

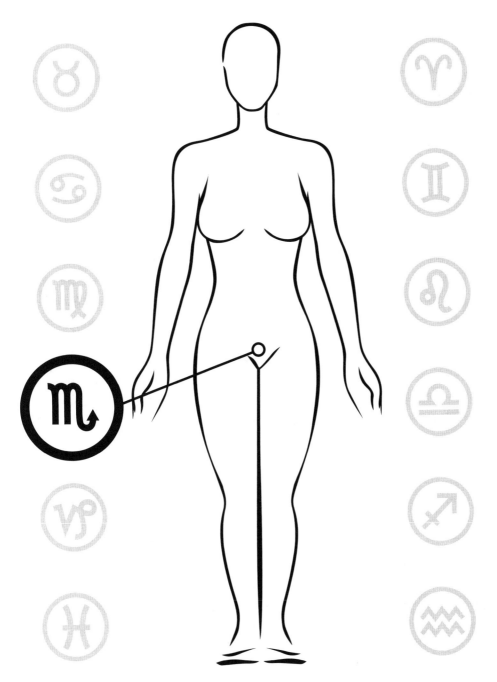

See appendix C for the skeletal structure of the sacrum.

In addition to the reproductive contents of the pelvic basin are urinary ones, like the bladder. Altogether, they make the region a highly fluid one; Scorpio is a water sign, so this may come as no surprise. In fact, astrologically speaking, the region's fluidity is simply the physical representation of a sign that is all about containment of emotion. Water and fluids in the area flow at both gross and molecular levels. This flow is like that of emotions, which move you toward your likes (such as your favorite restaurant) and away from your dislikes (such as rats). So fluid, flow, emotions, and motion are related, and the fluid-filled sacral center is thereby considered your body's seat of movement and sensation.

♏ Interestingly, the movement-related properties of emotions are embedded in the very word: *emotion* derives from the Latin *emovere*, with e- meaning "out of, utterly" and *movere* relating to movement. In other words, emotions move you out and about.

The Scorpio is a very passionate creature—she instinctively knows what she likes and does not like, and she draws a firm line between the two. She is prone to high highs and low lows, as water can reach a boil just as easily as it can turn to ice, which is why it is of utmost importance to focus on the region's balance and stability. Ideally, you want each side of your pelvis to be level and directed straight ahead, not tilted, rotated, or with one side higher than the other. In other words, you want to maintain a neutral pelvis, which will help stack your body above and below and also prevent sacroiliac joint discomfort and pain from misalignment. Developing and maintaining a neutral pelvis may take a lifetime of work, as it can be a difficult region to access.

The first step is to sense where your neutral pelvis is. Use this exercise to self-assess:

1. Lie on your back with knees bent and feet flat on the floor, about hip distance apart. Arms are elongated by your sides with palms facing down.
2. Place one hand between the curve of your lower back and the floor. Extend or flex your back—*just small movements are needed throughout this exercise*—so that there is just enough room for the width of your hand. This position should approximate your neutral pelvis.
3. Do an anterior tilt: tilt your pelvis forward—toward your knees—so that your lower back arches and there is excess space between your back, hand, and floor. This position is common in folks who have lordotic posture (see chapter 8: "Balance of the Scales").
4. Do a posterior tilt: engage your abdominal muscles to bring your pelvis back through neutral in order to tilt it the other direction, toward your head. Your

pelvis should tuck so that your lower back comes flat upon the floor and your hand is compressed between the two; your sitting bones should remain on the floor. A posterior tilt is a stable position for the back.

5. Return to your neutral position by subtly tilting your pelvis forward again. Sense how the position feels on the floor (which will be easier than when standing). Feel free to tilt between positions as much as necessary to establish your sense of a neutral pelvis.

6. Carefully stand up into what you consider your relaxed or normal stance. Can you sense how your pelvis is directed (neutral or tilted)? If it is tilted, make the necessary anterior or posterior adjustments to move your pelvis into neutral.

A neutral pelvis forms the foundation of your musculoskeletal world. It is the junction between the torso above and the lower limbs below. Its alignment, therefore, can either set a proper foundation for, or wreak havoc on, the rest of your form. Hence, the importance of its neutrality and stability. Given the extremes—the heights and depths—that Scorpios may experience, they can take care of themselves by keeping their sacral center in check.

> Antares is the star at the heart ♏ ♏
> of the Scorpio constellation.
> Its name means "like Ares"
> or "rivaling Ares" (referring
> to the Greek god of war).
> According to mythology,
> Orion wanted to kill all the
> animals on the planet, so the
> Earth goddess, Gaia, sent the
> scorpion to sting him. Both
> were subsequently placed
> in the sky, on opposite sides
> of the heavens, so that the
> strategic scorpion can keep
> the warrior in check.

The Stars: Scorpio

Die, Transform, and Soar

Death means different things to different people. To the Ancient Egyptians, it marked the end of life on Earth and—after a precarious journey through the underworld— an afterlife in a lush paradise. To the Aztecs death was an eternal sleep, and their region still celebrates an annual *Día de los Muertos* to honor those who came before. To many of us in Western society, it is an end to life as we know it, decomposition into dust, a finality to fight against or a gateway to heaven. In the context of Scorpio, death can be applied to any situation when letting go is necessary, when you are called to release a part of you that no longer belongs, like an expectation, personal baggage, or an old story.

You may recall that the Virgo similarly purifies parts of herself. This purification is driven by the desire to be a clear vessel for her service, so there is a perpetual pruning

♏ Fittingly, many of the world's celebrations of the dead fall within the month of Scorpio, including: the Mexican *Día de los Muertos*, the Celtic Samhain, the Catholic All Saints' Day, and the American Halloween.

process. Scorpio energy, in contrast, is here to purify for the purpose of catharsis, death, and rebirth. And so she lets go of all the underlying reasons for her patterns—the emotions, instincts, and drives that govern her daily thoughts and behaviors. In other words, Scorpio's death and destruction are outdated aspects of the id. Your id is a psychic force related to your sense of survival, safety, power, sex; it is the primal force underlying your thoughts and behaviors that desires immediate gratification. When mediated by other aspects of your consciousness, ego, and superego, your id allows you to satisfy basic urges like eating, drinking, and sleeping in a balanced way.

Each of us has a Scorpio who must confront aspects of the id that are out of balance—like a fear that is holding her back—in order to let go. She does not even need to know the specific aspects—she does not need to label them or understand through what complex interaction of self, school, family, society, media, and karma they arose. She just needs to know that it is time for parts of her that are no longer serving her highest purpose to die.

Death itself, then, becomes a process of great importance. It presents the ultimate way to connect to and govern the underworkings of your very nature. And to allow for a lifetime of learning, death must occur again and again. As with Persephone, the fair maiden in Greek mythology who dies to be reborn every year, thereby allowing the seasons to cycle: Spring occurs when she is on the planet's surface with her mother, Demeter, but winter comes every time she dies and returns to the underworld and her husband Hades (Pluto in Roman mythology, which also happens to be Scorpio's ruling planet). When your Scorpio metaphorically dies, she remains on the surface of Earth but as a new incarnation of herself. Her death is frequently catalyzed by some form of upheaval—like a near-death experience, financial ruin, or a loss of family—from which she is thrust from the old and into the new. And while these cataclysmic scenarios might not be intentionally executed, your Scorpio nature may subconsciously attract situations full of chaos and crisis *in order to die*. Because they are a part of the sign's very fabric. These challenging situations are the way that the universe teaches you to release old attachments, which is why the situations will appear again and again—to help you accept death, learn from it, and ultimately, teach others its wisdom.

Death has a stigma in our society. But it is only as bad as we have made it. Otherwise, it is what it is, neither good nor bad. Rather, it is a process to be respected and learned from; one so fundamental to life that no one should go without its metaphysical process occurring multiple times. Just like the scorpion arachnid dies about six times—molting its exoskeleton—in order to be fully formed. It is a literal and figurative shedding of old skin that precipitates change. For the zodiac's Scorpio, though, what comes after death is secondary to the sacred and profound process of death itself. Death connects you with you at your deepest, scariest, most primordial level. It offers the chance to see, accept, and act upon parts of yourself, however you might need to. It is truly a great gift that Scorpio brings—an inner alchemy that allows you to turn into gold what used to be lead.

Alchemy was an ancient mystical protoscience—a precursor to modern chemistry and medicine—whose central tenet rested around the philosopher's stone, an elusive substance that was believed to turn lead into gold. While the stone was thought to be a type of salt, it was believed to be the key ingredient in the pursuit of immortality, enlightenment, and heaven-on-earth bliss. It symbolized, therefore, our own transformation from not only one element to another but also from mortal to divine.

Our society loves a good transformation story. Children read tales of how a frog turns into prince, teens see movies showing Clark Kent morphing into Superman, and adults pick up magazines with before and after photos. This fixation belies a fascination with underlying potential, with recognition of what can be as opposed to what currently is. Transformation is what allows you to move through internal and external attachments that keep you imprisoned and enslaved, to grow into a new version of who you are and how you live, or as the Scorpio artist Pablo Picasso put it, "Different motives inevitably require different methods of expression."[1]

Within Plato's *Timaeus*, his inadvertent astrology text, he describes a *prima materia* (first matter) from which all substance is made. *Prima materia* is also the name that ancient alchemists assigned to the starting ingredient for the philosopher's stone.

Easier said than done, for transformation is no easy feat. In fact, it is uncomfortable and unfamiliar. The mind does not like it at all—for even if you dislike your current box, you still may prefer it to one that is unknown. At any given time, the mind would prefer to hold on to your current construct of self than let you expand or exchange it.

To successfully change therefore implies resilience, a form of faith that you can bounce back and recover from whatever adversity you may face. This quality is one that your inner Scorpio possesses in spades, as long as you are willing to let go and allow transformation to occur, not sure of where it will take you. Hence, any good transformation is like its precursor, death, in that it exacts a need for respect and trust in the process.

If your Scorpio side holds on to who you currently are and what you have got, she will subvert the deep, mysterious chaos that is her birthright, and then she will become stuck. Reinvention will be replaced by resistance, and inner chaos will not be channeled into internal transformation—but external control. As this occurs so will manipulation of others, a less evolved way for the Scorpio to meet what she perceives as her end goals (especially in areas concerning wealth and sex). It is therefore of supreme importance that we embrace our Scorpio side and help her embrace her inner chaos, her drive to transform. She must be willing to be a phoenix that does not necessarily know to what heights it will rise after it burns. Only that she will rise to soar, time and again.

To soar is to rise above it all, to view a situation from its greatest context and meaning, above the thoughts, emotions, trifles, and tribulations that are otherwise present. Mind you, a Scorpio's calm and collected demeanor is often just the still water under which the torrents rage. But to be at her most evolved, soaring provides a poignant reminder to keep her raw nature—her id—controlled. To engage in a cool mastery that belies the dynamic power inside. That way, she can see what she wants and obtain it with calculated precision—like the way an eagle, from high in the sky, will quickly and accurately home in on a field mouse to satisfy its instinctual hunger before it ascends again.

The eagle represents the highest stage of Scorpio. Scorpio may actually be symbolized by three different animals: the Scorpion, the Phoenix, and the Eagle. The Scorpion is related to the death drive, the Phoenix to transformation, and the Eagle to soaring. It is a cycle of death and rebirth that enables the Scorpio to be, do, and get what she wants—a tremendous power that she needs to be aware of in order to maintain discipline, lest she find herself under its control.

♏ A great example of unbridled id is that of Mr. Hyde—the darker, lascivious nature of the otherwise good Dr. Jekyll. *The Strange Case of Dr. Jekyll and Mr. Hyde* is a tale of inner duality in which the darkness wins, penned by the Scorpio author Robert Louis Stevenson. It is believed that during the writing process, he burned the first draft of his story only to rewrite the current version, which figuratively rose from the ashes.

Lessons

Scorpio's power and passion make her bankrupt one day and a billionaire the next. In this way, she shows that no matter what is going on, you can die and be reborn. It is the zodiac's reminder of your power of transformation and resilience—the part of you that can be and do anything at any time, even if you are currently going up in flames. Or down. After all, the Scorpio's emotions range from mountain peaks to valleys.

To use the depth of your Scorpio emotions constructively requires that you control them and channel them so you can harness their power and not be destroyed by it. Of course, there are many times when you need to metaphorically die, but if you get stuck in the death stage you will never reach transformation . . . and then never soar.

Getting stuck is a downfall of this sign's energy—just as water stagnates, so does our Scorpio nature if she becomes attached to old stories, instincts, and fears. And then muck accrues. So she must learn from each of her deaths; otherwise she will not be able to move on. She will continue to be the person she was and is, never progressing to the person she needs to be.

Physical manifestations of a stagnant Scorpio nature may include:

★ Tight, contracted muscles of the lower back, hamstrings, abdomen, gluteal region, or pelvic floor at their attachments on the sacrum or pelvis
★ Ache or discomfort in the lower back or gluteal region
★ Restricted range of motion of the lower back or pelvis
★ A fixed, non-neutral pelvis (e.g., one side higher than the other)
★ Other: Menstrual cycle irregularity, urinary retention

Similarly, when your Scorpio is not in balance—whether physically, emotionally, or otherwise—your sacral region may experience a sensation of feeling out of whack or out of place, due to extremes. In this scenario, it may feel as loose or uncontrolled as you do.

Physical manifestations of a loose Scorpio nature may include:

★ Weak and potentially elongated muscles of the lower back, hamstrings, abdomen, gluteal region, or pelvic floor that are unable to maintain the proper placement of the sacrum or pelvis
★ Sensation of weakness or instability in the pelvic region

★ Hypermobility

★ Excess pelvic rotation, flare, or tilt

★ Other: Menstrual cycle irregularity, urinary tract infection, incontinence due to weak pelvic floor muscles (Weak pelvic floor muscles may occur with age or post-pregnancy, after the Scorpio opens into the role of mother—along with the bones, muscles, and ligaments of her pelvis. See the Kegel exercise in this chapter as a means of pelvic floor maintenance and problem prevention.)

How sensitive is your sacral center? Whether it feels stagnant, loose, or somewhere in between, the key is listening to your body and giving it what it needs. To stretch a tight sacral center or strengthen a weak one, awaken your inner Scorpio with the questions and exercises that follow.

Your Body and the Stars

The following will serve as your personal guide to embodying the story of the Scorpio stars. Use them to die, transform, and soar.

Questions

★ What are your beliefs around death? How do they help your life? Hinder it?

★ How well are you able to let go of past attachments, expectations?

★ When is the last time that you reinvented yourself? What precipitated this death and rebirth?

★ When was the last time you experienced discomfort in any part of your sacral center? What was occurring in your life?

★ How readily do you acclimate to new surroundings and transform? Is it a process that you welcome or fight?

★ How many emotions do you feel during the course of a week? Do you access your full emotional range?

★ When you experience negative emotional extremes, are you able to rise above them? How?

★ When you experience positive extremes, what circumstances bring you back down?

Exercises

Bridge Pose: For Strength to Let Go

Death—even at the metaphysical level—is just one stage in the progression of consciousness. It is not good or bad, but only as you make it. You may approach it with fear or, equally, with an open mind as to where it will take you. The key is to allow it to take you there, allowing your fear of death to die in the process. To do so, release whatever stigma you have placed around it. Harness the power in you that knows—despite not knowing what comes on the other side of the bridge—you will be all right. That death's natural flow will take you where you need to go. It takes strength to trust this unknown process and cross the bridge. Cultivate inner strength through the strength of your sacral center and muscles surrounding it.

1. Lie on your back, with your knees bent and feet flat on the floor. Arms are elongated by your sides with palms facing down. Place your feet in front of your sitting bones—a good distance will allow you to brush your fingertips upon your heels.
2. On an exhale, press your feet into the floor as you tuck your pelvis (your lower back will flatten on the floor). Continuing with the same momentum, raise your buttocks. Only your feet, arms, shoulders, neck, and head should now be on the floor.
3. Within the pose, keep your thighs and feet parallel. Extend through the arms to help you stay on your shoulders. Create space between your chin and chest by gently pressing the back of your head into the floor. Relax your buttocks; they should be active but not gripping.
4. Remain in the pose for ten breaths. Release on an exhalation, slowly rolling your spine down along the floor.

If maintaining a raised back and buttocks is challenging, keep your arms on the ground, bend your elbows, and raise your forearms to place your hands on your lower back for extra support (fingers pointing toward toes). You may also use yoga blocks for even more help. If you feel stable in the pose and desire further release, maintain your foundation and rotate only your forearms so that your palms face up, in a position of openness to whatever comes next.

Cat-Cow: To Transform

Scorpio is believed to be one of the more intuitive signs. More in touch with her inner magic, mystery, and alchemy. So be your own philosopher's stone and practice changing parts of yourself from lead into gold. Turn shame into joy, hunger to satiety, "I can't" to "I can." Yours is a long life during which many changes will occur and, as they say, chance favors the prepared. Prepare for your inevitable transformations by practicing with this popular pose, which will give you the chance to transform from a cat to a cow (and back again).

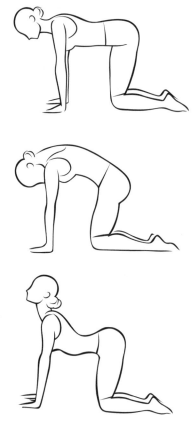

1. Start in a tabletop position on your hands and knees, with wrists under shoulders and knees under hips. Tops of your feet are flat on the floor. Your back is parallel to the floor, and your neck is neutral, with the gaze down on the floor and slightly in front of you.
2. Enter into cat: On an exhale, round your spine toward the ceiling. Press your hands and feet into the floor to help the lift. As your back rounds, gently release your head toward the floor.
3. Enter into cow: On the following inhale, lift your sitting bones and arch your chest toward the ceiling. Your belly will sink toward the floor. Your head should follow the upward arch of your spine, but be careful not to overextend your neck.
4. Return to cat pose on the subsequent exhale, then cow on the inhale. Create a rhythmic flow as you move between the two.
5. Cycle through ten rounds of cat-cow, ending in tabletop position.

Release the pose into child's pose (see page 89 for child's pose instructions).

Reclining Bound Angle Pose: To Access Your Depths

Your sacral center is home to your sexuality, both in terms of your sexual organs and you as a sexual being. But few folks have a healthy relationship with sexuality, as many Anglo-European countries have culturally, religiously, and medically denied, negated, and even viewed it as evil for centuries.

Displeasure with sexuality reached a defining moment in the eighteenth century when physicians declared that masturbation needed to be controlled for hygiene and medical reasons. Otherwise, they claimed that a weakening of the digestive, respiratory, and nervous systems might result, as might sterility, rheumatism, gonorrhea, blindness, insanity, and tumors. From that time on, circumcision (initially performed on boys, not babies) became one of the more popular medical procedures of the day.

This region of your body is even referred to as your "nether regions," which connotes the lowest and darkest parts of a place, with a special allusion to hell and the underworld. Reclaim this valid and valuable piece of you! Every part of you retains its own power, and your sexual region is no different. Use this pose to open into your fullest extent and access some depths that you might be unwittingly dismissing.

1. Sit with your legs straight out in front of you. Bend your knees and bring your heels toward your pelvis. As your heels come closer, drop your knees out to the sides in order to bring the soles of your feet together.
2. Lower your torso back down to the floor, using your forearms and hands for support.
3. Once your torso is on the floor, find a comfortable distance between your feet and pelvis (decrease or increase the distance for more or less stretch, respectively). This is a passive stretch, so you should feel a gentle opening in your groin area; if the stretch is too intense or there is pain in your knees, place cushions between your knees and the floor. Bring your palms to rest gently upon your lower abdomen.
4. Close your eyes and relax completely. Surrender into the pose. Allow gravity to do the work. Stay in the pose for five to ten minutes.
5. To exit the pose, press your thighs together as you roll over onto one side. Then slowly lift yourself up to prevent any lightheadedness.

To subtly deepen the pose, extend your tailbone isometrically toward your feet. You should feel a gentle engagement and opening of the sacral center as well as a slight arch of the lower back. From this position, now allow your tailbone to sink into the floor.

Kundalini Visualization: To Soar

There is more than one way to skin a cat . . . and elevate a snake. In terms of awakening your Kundalini—the metaphorical serpent residing at the base of your spine and representing your instinctual life force—the journey can take many different forms depending on your level of commitment, intention behind it, current level of consciousness, and lifestyle. In most forms, however, the journey involves the ascent of the serpent up your spine and out the top of your head. The following exercise offers a visualization of the ascent, as the serpent—and the subconscious life force it represents—can many times be better grasped through images and archetypes than through words or thoughts.

What does it feel like when your Kundalini rises? Its awakening involves many sensations, some of which have been likened to currents of electricity running through your body, divine bliss, and a feeling of lightness—as if your earthly form could soar. This exercise is not intended to fully awaken your Kundalini but to help you peek into its potential and prepare.

1. Sit comfortably in a cross-legged position on the floor. Maintain a straight and relaxed spine. Palms are facing up while resting on your lap. Eyes are closed.
2. In your mind's eye, visualize a serpent coiled three and a half times around the area of your sacrum. Give it color, eyes, scales—any form you choose. The more detailed, the better. Inhale and exhale to greet it.
3. As if pulled by some magnetic force from the top of your head, let the serpent arise and *slowly* travel up your spine. Take an inhale and exhale at each of the following regions as it moves through them: sacral center (between navel and groin), abdomen (around the navel), heart center, middle of the throat, third eye, top of the head. Feel the sensation in each body region as it travels there.
4. As it starts exiting the top of your head, watch as both you and the serpent merge and explode into a bright white light. Feel the sensation of the light for as long as possible.
5. Open your eyes and pause before arising.

If you want to fully awaken your Kundalini, consider personal guidance through the resources of Kundalini yoga.

Incorporate Water: For Emotions, Movement, and Flow

Let water allow your emotions to flow. You have a whole spectrum of sensations available to you, and they all serve a purpose—even maligned ones like anger, which can catalyze positive change at individual and societal levels. Very few people who have transformed the world did it because they were okay with the status quo! So let yourself rise to great heights and fall to great lows. In other words, live with passion. Do not get stuck in a comfortable range of emotion, but be willing and able to expand it. Incorporate water into your daily routine to let its tides inspire yours:

* ★ Take a walk by a river, lake, or ocean
* ★ Be deliberate about drinking pure, filtered water throughout the day
* ★ Turn the routine of a shower into an enjoyable ritual
* ★ Go swimming
* ★ Take off your shoes and frolic in a water fountain
* ★ Go to a water park and have fun

Kegel Exercise: For Proper Containment

When water is channeled—whether from a tributary into a river or from the faucet into a glass—it serves its purpose best. The same is true for your emotions too. Released emotions require a conduit or container. Otherwise, they may run willy-nilly, and havoc (followed by fatigue) will ensue. Give your emotions a proper form so that they can fuel you, not inadvertently leak out from you. One form is with a strong pelvic bowl, which supports its fluid-related sacral contents (namely the bladder and the uterus). Some of the bowl's muscles can be readily accessed—like the deep lateral rotators that are stretched in the reclining bound angle pose—but others, like the muscles of the pelvic floor, are not so easy to reach. One of the best ways to strengthen them is through Kegel exercises, beneficial for both men and women.

1. Identify the proper muscles. Engage the pelvic floor muscles by arresting urination in midstream. This action uses the same muscles that the Kegels engage.
2. Practice Kegel contractions. The Kegel exercise is exactly the same technique you used to stop urination—but not while you are urinating. Empty your bladder and then lie on your back. Contract your pelvic floor muscles

as you did earlier and hold the contraction for ten seconds. Then relax for ten seconds. This is one set.

3. Concentrate only on the pelvic floor, and do not contract other muscles like your buttocks, abdomen, or thighs. Remember to breathe.

4. Repeat three sets up to three times a day. You may also perform them while seated in an upright position.

These exercise are believed to help prevent urinary incontinence and may even help improve sexual health and pleasure.

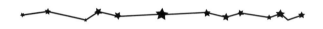

Summary

★ Your sacral center is the region related to Scorpio. Home to the reproductive organs and womb, it represents the seed of life and seat of emotions.

★ Scorpio is the eighth sign of the zodiac cycle. Its energy pertains to a passion that drives you to metaphorically die, transform, and then rise again.

★ If your powerful Scorpio nature becomes either stagnated or out of control, your sacral center might experience different symptoms (e.g., sacroiliac discomfort, menstrual irregularities).

★ Invoke your inner Scorpio through questions, exercises, and activities that focus on your sacral center. Use them to rise above inner strife and outer turmoil, to regain a greater worldview that allows you to soar.

Note
1. "Conversation avec Picasso," by Christian Zervos, Cathiers d'Art: 1935, quoted and translated in Alfred H. Barr, Jr., *Picasso: Fifty Years of His Art* (New York: The Museum of Modern Art, 1946), 247.

10

Hips of the Centaur

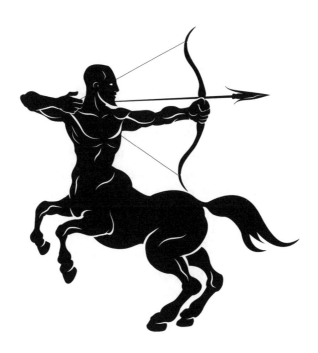

♐ SAGITTARIUS

Birth date: November 22–December 21
Body region: Hips and Thighs
Theme: Direct Your Lower Nature
with Higher Aspiration

With Sagittarius, we exit the zodiac's tour of the upper body and focus on the lower body, starting at the hips. Of course, the body operates as a unified whole, so this upper-lower divide is in name only. But the lesson of the Centaur is to consciously align the two and what they represent. For the Sagittarius is here to evolve the body as a vehicle for the soul, helping you aspire to living your highest, purest ideals as a twenty-four-hour-a-day goal.

Your Body: Hips and Thighs

Whatever his journey, the Centaur receives his lessons and help from his hips, the region of the body corresponding to the Sagittarian sign. Perfectly poised for the Sagittarian struggle, these two large joints are juxtaposed between the upper and lower body. The upper body reaches from the pelvis toward the head and includes the intervening back, neck, upper limbs, and internal organs (collectively referred to as the trunk); the lower body extends downward from the pelvis, encompassing the thighs, legs, and feet. You can feel your hips deeply set on each side of your loins, the depth of these joints a source of their physical strength.

> ↗ The region of the pelvis, hips, and thighs provides the closest example within the body of where a human torso would arise from the hindquarters of a horse, thereby forming a centaur.

Strong hips are formed from strong bones, including the pelvis and femur. The pelvis is a wide, bony basin that supports the weight of the trunk above, and transfers its force to the limbs below. It is one of the bones that, by virtue of its position in the body, enables humans to stand erect on two feet, an anatomical trait distinguishing us from the rest of our vertebrate brethren, including horses (read more in chapter 13: "Feet of the Fish"). As part of the hip joint, the pelvis provides a deep socket into which the head of the femur fits. The femur is the thighbone, the longest bone in the body. Its head is a round, shiny ball that settles into the pelvis's socket. Together, these two bones form a type of joint known as a ball-and-socket.

> ↗ Many individuals mistakenly locate their hips on the side of each thigh. This location is actually a bony prominence on the femur called the greater trochanter. It is, therefore, part of a bone that comprises the hip joint but not the joint itself.

The ball-and-socket joint of the hip moves the region of the thigh. Each thigh extends from the pelvis to the knee and, especially in Sagittarians, is a well-formed part of the body—robust and ready to leap right into the action. The thigh's range of movements is as expansive as its zodiac sign: flexion, extension, abduction, adduction, and rotation. These movements—taken alone or in combination—facilitate many daily actions, from stepping to stampeding. Flexion,

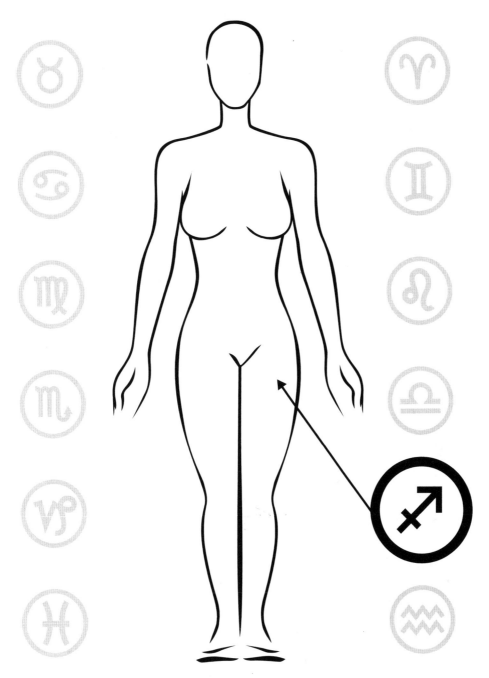

See appendix C for the skeletal structure of the hips and thighs.

for example, is the movement that starts any step or stampede, raising the thigh closer to the front of the body so you can pick your foot up off the ground and head forth on your inner Centaur's journey.

Wherever your journey takes you—whether to the airport or an ashram—your hips help move you there. But where is *there*? Where are you off to explore? To get where you want requires not only movement but also direction. Herein lies the life-work of every Centaur—he must pursue a direction, and his path calls for him to choose the highest one—the one that fulfills him body-and-soul. And while this inspired undertaking is not easy for anyone, it's even harder for the zodiac signs whose tendency is toward the lower.

For a body to bear forth soul, he must, therefore, align the upper with the lower half; he must dream of being a professor for his hips to move him through the school's front doors. More than metaphysics, this upper-lower alignment is physical reality. Experience it for yourself:

1. Stand straight and find a neutral position for your pelvis, with hips pointed squarely ahead.
2. Above your pelvis, align head over shoulders, shoulders over torso, and torso over hips. Below your pelvis, align hips over knees and knees over ankles and feet.
3. Choose a point of focus several feet in front of you.
4. Walk toward it.

How did you get there? With head, chest, and hips aligned, you walked decisively in the direction of your choosing. You had a vision of what you wanted, and you reached it. In contrast, what happens when you lack this alignment?

1. Stand straight, with your hips pointed squarely ahead.
2. Maintaining the position of your pelvis and lower limbs, rotate your head and chest to the left. Your hips and lower limbs should now be facing one direction (straight) and your torso another (left).
3. Walk forward.

In which direction did you go? In this example, you did not choose a direction, and your body defaulted to the one provided by its lower half. You went the way your hips were positioned—a physical example of the susceptibility of every Centaur toward his lower leanings.

The Stars: Sagittarius

Direct Your Lower Nature with Higher Aspiration

Sagittarius is Latin for "archer" and the symbol for its constellation is, fittingly, an arrow. This arrow is directed by the Centaur, half-man half-beast, who aims it into the sky toward broad horizons. With the pluck of his bow, he shoots the arrow, blazing a fiery trail for his bold journey ahead—a journey that calls for the Sag to direct his body toward the urgings of his soul.

There are many ways to direct yourself, whether you are wondering what food to eat or what job to take. Direction can come through rational thought, emotional attraction, gut instincts, or some combination of these and more. It can arise from you or from others. How do you choose your direction in life? There is no right or wrong direction—only the one that serves you best. Your true direction is the one that comes from your true nature, from a place of knowing that is filtered through the mind but is also greater. It is that subtle sense of purpose—as if your soul came into this lifetime with a mission to fulfill—that you glimpse every now and then. Your Sagittarius is here to acknowledge that glimpse, to induce you to trust it, and then to help you follow its direction . . . wherever it leads.

For the Centaur is your inner pathfinder, visionary, guide. It's the part of you that implicitly senses your grand direction and inspires you to aim for it again and again. Sometimes you hit your target on the first attempt, and sometimes you must shoot many arrows. You do not need to know how the arrow will get to its goal—or if it will—but the first step to get there is to know where *there* is. To hit a specific target, your sights cannot be too high or too low.

Low is a term that comes with a stigma in our society as if it is bad or undesirable. And yet, all *low* really means is "toward the ground or base level," as when the moon sits low on the horizon, not a particularly debasing definition. *High*, its counterpart, pertains to an elevated status, as an eagle flies high in the sky. Of course, it is all relative, so that even things that are high in the sky can be low relative to others and vice versa—just like a high-flying eagle is still lower than a low-set moon. This is because high and low qualities exist in tandem. They complement each other. One is not better than the other, as both are necessary.

For instance, you have both lower and higher natures. In terms of our energetic makeup, our lower nature refers to the part that is denser than the rest, like our physical body (versus spirit) or thoughts that are base (versus illumined). Low goals only become a problem if they lead your life story, if you overly consume yourself with basic wants and needs without acknowledging the part of you that is simultaneously greater. At one extreme, catering to only your low nature may result in the proverbial life of sex, drugs, and rock and roll, with desire leading to dissatisfying relationships, ambition to money's meaningless success, and excess to inconspicuous consumption. Low begets lower is a story for the ages, a moral written in the stars of the Sagittarian Centaur....

Once upon a time—according to Greek mythology—centaurs roamed the earth. These liminal creatures, half man and half horse, lived in the mountains of Magnesia. They made homes in caves, hunted wild animals for food, and fought with rocks and branches. Throughout classical Greek and Roman works—from Homer's *Odyssey* to Ovid's *The Metamorphoses*—these centaurs typified man's most primitive tendencies as they pillaged towns, stole women, and downed more wine than Dionysus (the Greek god of the vine). Their raw, savage attributes were embodied in their beastly hindquarters, resembling the rear end of a horse and representing man's most animalistic aspects. But their cautionary tale is only half of the story, for these creatures were also human. Each centaur had a human torso rising from its equine body—a head, neck, and chest, epitomizing man's loftiest ideals.

Just as the first breed of centaurs were slaves to their animalistic, lower natures, there roamed another breed of centaur who honored their higher, human aspects. Those who were teachers and healers, who wielded wisdom and prophetic vision. One such centaur was named Chiron, a friend and teacher to the great warrior Hercules. One day, while helping Hercules, Chiron was wounded by a poisoned arrow. Zeus, as a gift to the good centaur, relieved his pain by turning him into the constellation Sagittarius. The Centaur thus became the zodiac symbol for the Sagittarian sign, symbolizing the highest nature of man.

Like the Centaur, you have both higher and lower natures that reside together. To live the fullest expression of you requires that you access *both* halves—and this is where honoring your inner Sagittarius can help. Otherwise, too much of either side creates a life out of balance. In our society, with our focus on food and finances, the tendency is toward the lower nature. So your Sagittarius nature is a reminder that to be a complete you, you need to access your creativity, vision, imagination, and intuition in addition to your lower drives. You need to stand firmly on the ground *and* aim for the stars.

The juxtaposition between high and low plays into Sagittarian author John Milton's most famous seventeenth-century works, *Paradise Lost* and *Paradise Regained*. *Paradise Lost* tells the story of Satan's expulsion from heaven and his orchestration of Adam and Eve's fall from grace. Its sequel, *Paradise Regained*, recounts Jesus's temptation by and resistance to Satan and how he thereby passed the test—on behalf of all humanity—that Adam and Eve had originally failed.

Aiming for the stars is akin to setting your sights on something that seems beyond your current reach . . . until you get there! Which is what the Sagittarian engineer Alexandre Gustave Eiffel did after constructing the Eiffel Tower, the tallest building in the world (at the time): he entered the field of aerodynamics and developed subsequent structures—like planes—that not just extended into the sky but also could fly. This high aim is aspiration, a chief motivating force of the Centaur.

The evolved Centaur is an idealist, a visionary who sees beyond what is to what is possible. And that glimpse into the infinite potential is what fuels his continuous journey forward. There is always room to grow and evolve in order to be better in your various roles as parent, professional, and person.

Of course, you do not have to aspire. Heck, you are free to tread water, or even regress. But true Sag energy aims toward the highest ideal possible. The ideal does not have to be reached—nor may it even be possible—but that is the drive. Or gallop, rather, since the Centaur is blessed with four fast-moving hooves (although a horse's hoof is actually its single toe).

The origin of the word *aspire* comes from the Latin *aspirare*, with *a* referring to "to" and *spirare* to "breathe," a root that also encompasses *spiri*, which denotes "spirit." Aspire may, then, also mean "to breathe in spirit."

What do you aspire to be or do in your life? What heights are you moving toward? The awesome thing about aspiration is that it is only possible to see so high . . . and to assume what waits for you there. You cannot possibly know for sure until you are there to experience it for yourself. Once you get there, it inevitably looks different than you might have envisioned it. And then you realize it is not the ultimate height for you to reach but merely a way station en route to another spire that you can only now see.

And so the process continues, for aspiration is not about having reached great heights but about continually reaching for them. And as we are living in a universe of one hundred billion observed galaxies (and growing), the height of your reach is poised to expand.

Lessons

The direction the Centaur walks has to align with the directions of his upper and lower halves. In this way, he unifies his natures. He allows his lower nature (represented by his lower limbs) to bring to life his highest ideals and heartfelt aspirations (represented by his head and heart).

If he is successful in this venture, the Sag will feel fulfilled. He will be living a balanced life, attending to all aspects of himself—lower, higher, and everything in between. The tendency, however, is for your Sag nature to be susceptible to his lower tendencies, to the gluttony and desire that he will want to voraciously fulfill. But this is what he is here to learn and, ultimately, teach: how to take control of your lower, animalistic nature with the discipline, compromise, and intuition necessary to hear and heed his divinity.

> ↗ Recognize gluttony and overpowering desire? According to the catechism of the Catholic Church, they are the first two of the seven deadly sins, which are the origin of all others. They are "deadly" because this consumption by the lower nature of man is believed to destroy grace and charity—aspects of his higher nature—and thereby lead to eternal damnation.

If the direction of the lower becomes so incongruent with the upper, the hips reflect this metaphysical burden and fall from physical alignment too. Through a variety of musculoskeletal aches and pains, they will prevent your trajectory forward by making your journey a struggle. This is their way of letting you know, "Hey, you're not moving in the best direction for you, so we refuse to let you keep heading there." If, for example, you are moving in a direction that does not serve your highest purpose, your hips will sound an alert. In this scenario, it is likely that they will be tight and restricted, as your inner Centaur tries to prevent you from charging ahead on a path that is not necessarily your best—despite your best intentions. Or you may have chosen a path that is indeed your calling, but the way in which you are pursuing it—too quickly or aggressively—results in your hips registering the incongruence. Part of your Centurion journey requires faith in divine timing. Faith that what you want and need to occur will, in due time (which, is not always aligned with your mind's sense of time). Otherwise, you will find yourself grumbling about best-laid plans with a hint of self-righteous indignation.

Physical manifestations of a righteous Sagittarius energy may include:

★ Tight or strained hip muscles (e.g., flexors or extensors)
★ Imbalanced hip muscles (e.g., abductors)
★ Fixed internal or external rotation of thighs
★ Limited range of hip motion
★ Iliotibial band tightness
★ Pain felt at the joints, around the greater trochanters or gluteal region
★ Nerve pain in the gluteal region or back of the thigh
★ Other: Over-indulgence in food or drink, liver imbalance

Conversely, if your Sagittarian self is unwilling to take the horse by the reins and commit to a course, you will also find yourself out of sorts. Unbridled interests will shift from here to there, but you will never commit your vast energy to one direction. In other words, this reckless aspect of your nature will encourage you to go everywhere and try everything—without contemplation. You will be wildly and impractically aiming your bow. Or, perhaps you aim well but lack follow-through as multiple directions compete for your attention. Given many opportunities, you might feel paralyzed in choosing, or not believe that there is a direction worth your while and so you do everything but your direction as you wait for a destination to somehow arrive for you. On the part of the archer, these examples might result in hips that do not know where to go.

Physical manifestations of a reckless Sagittarius energy may include:

★ Weak hip muscles (e.g., flexors or extensors)
★ Imbalanced hip muscles (e.g., abductors)
★ Hypermobility of hip joints
★ Excessive internal or external rotation of thighs
★ Iliotibial band tightness
★ Non-neutral pelvic position (see chapter 9: "Sacrum of the Scorpio")
★ Nerve pain in the gluteal region or back of the thigh
★ Other: Over-indulgence in food or drink, liver imbalance

How committed are your hips to your direction? Whether they feel righteous, reckless, or somewhere in between, the key is listening to your body and giving it what it needs. To stretch tight hips or strengthen weak ones, awaken your inner Sagittarius with the questions and exercises that follow.

Your Body and the Stars

The following will serve as your personal guide to embodying the story of the Sagittarius stars. Use them to direct your lower nature with your highest aspirations.

Questions

- ★ How would you describe your current direction in life?
- ★ Is your current direction the one you ideally envision for yourself? If so, to what do you attribute your success in this regard? If not, what steps could you take to change course?
- ★ What do your hips say about your sense of direction? Are they strong, weak, open?
- ★ What aspects of your higher and lower natures could be brought into better balance (for example, eating or drinking too much, staying up too late)?
- ★ What activities evoke your higher nature?
- ★ To what do you aspire? At the end of your life, how do you wish to be remembered?

Exercises

Chair Pose: For a Strong Sense of Direction

Direction can be hard to ascertain because it is not nearly as obvious or self-evident as one would like. Unlike signs on the road you drive, signs on the road of your life are not observable. Sure, clues are there, but they are subtle and easily missed . . . or dismissed. So knowing your life's direction and confidently following it can take faith and perseverance. Sort of like shooting a bow and arrow the first time: the whole business may feel clumsy and futile as your arrows keep falling from your bow or firing on a trajectory different than expected. But if you persist in your efforts, you will eventually be able to shoot an arrow in the direction of your mark. And hey, you might even land a bull's-eye! So proceed with determination. Use this exercise to strengthen the majority of the musculature surrounding your hip joints, as strong hips help confer a strong sense of direction. (Note that *tight* is not the same thing as *strong*. Hip flexors greatly benefit from diligent strengthening and stretching, as they become chronically short and tight in contemporary society, which is currently structured to maintain prolonged sitting positions in couches, office chairs, kitchen stools, and cars.)

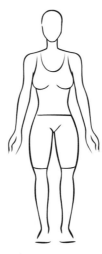

1. Stand with your feet hip distance apart. Bend your hips and knees on an exhale, lowering your thighs, as if sitting on a chair. Your thighs should be parallel to the floor, or the closest you are able to come to it with a neutral (not overly curved or extended) spine.

2. Inhale and elevate your arms next to your ears, with palms facing in, toward each other. If this position is uncomfortable, lower your arms and join your palms together in front of your heart.

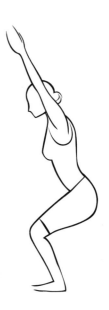

3. Ensure that your thighs are parallel to each other and that each knee is directed over the corresponding second toe. Your trunk will angle slightly forward over the thighs, and your neck and head should remain in line with the rest of your spine.

4. Maintain the position for five breath cycles. Release it by straightening your hips and knees on an inhalation and lowering your arms on the subsequent exhalation.

If this pose causes you to lose balance or feel weak or unstable, modify it by performing it with your back against a wall.

Pigeon Pose: To Open to Your Inner Direction

For about three thousand years, pigeons have been used to deliver messages. Whether in wartime to relay classified information or in ancient Greece to proclaim the winner of the Olympics, pigeons were used as reliable messengers due to their sense of direction. While they are not expert map readers, they do have an innate sense of home, which allows them to determine their location relative to their nest, to which they will always return. This same sense resides within you—the sense that your true direction is within, waiting

Homing pigeons were frequently employed by police departments in remote areas of India to deliver emergency news following natural disasters. It was not until recently that the Police Pigeon Service messenger system was retired (in favor of the internet).

to be discovered, and once you find it you will feel at home no matter where in the world you are. Use this pigeon pose to open your hips, and you'll open into a deeper understanding of direction that you might have not accessed before.

1. Start in a tabletop position on your hands and knees, with wrists under shoulders and knees under hips.

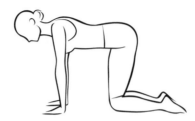

2. Extend the spine slightly to help lift the right thigh and flex the right knee. Slide the right leg forward and parallel to the top of the exercise mat so that the right knee comes behind the right wrist and the right foot comes toward the left wrist.
3. With the outside of the right leg resting on the floor, slide the left leg straight back by extending the left knee.
4. Lower the right sitting bone to the floor— without rolling onto your outer buttock—and place the top of the left foot on the floor.
5. The torso is straight, with the palms planted firmly on the floor either in front of the knees or next to each hip, depending on your ability. Maintain a neutral pelvis by adjusting the left side so it moves toward the front of the mat and in line with the right side.
6. Remain in this position for five slow, deep breaths.
7. Exit the pose by returning to the tabletop position.
8. Repeat on the left side.

This stretch is notoriously deep. If you would like to make it even deeper, lay your torso on the ground, extending the arms forward. Conversely, for a decreased stretch, decrease the angle of the front knee (drawing the foot closer toward the body), or place a cushion under the sitting bone of the front hip. Remember that your focus should be on proper alignment. Greater depth will occur naturally with practice and time.

Hip Circles: To Change Directions

The hip joints are almost as mobile as the shoulder joints, enabling a range of motion that effectively allows your hips and thighs to make full circles. From fan kicking to Hula-Hooping, your hips were designed to move in multiple directions. So do not become fixed on only one direction—do not focus so exclusively on your end destination that you lose focus on whether it is truly right for you. Within the course of your lifetime, you will change directions many times. So decide on your direction, but stay open to other opportunities that arise on the way there. Flexible hips acknowledge that any given direction is subject to change. Use these circles to create a general and gentle opening for the hip joints to allow your inner Sag to explore with ease.

> While Hula-Hoops reached popular prominence in the 1950s with the Wham-O company, they have been around since about 500 BCE. At that time, circles of willow or grapevines were used by Egyptian children to whirl around their waists. The ancient Greeks used similar hoops for exercise.

1. Stand up straight with your feet hip distance apart, feet grounded on the floor. Place your hands on your waist.
2. Slightly bend your knees and *gently* bounce up and down in this bend, settling into it. After a few bounces, keep your knees slightly bent.
3. With your torso facing front, circle your hips toward the right. Make the circles as large as you can without too much movement in the rest of your body, as if you were circling a Hula-Hoop. Your torso will shift a bit, but your knees should not buckle, your shoulders should remain even, and your head should not jut out.
4. Perform ten circles to the right and then ten to the left.

This exercise will open not only your hips but also your lower back. Smile! Allow yourself to open . . . and enjoy!

Reach for the Stars: For Aspiration

There are thought to be up to 400 billion stars in our galaxy (the Milky Way) alone. The closest star is the Sun at a mere 93 million miles . . . compared to the next closest stars of the Alpha Centauri system, which is approximately 4.3 light-years away (with one light-year equaling 5.9 x 10^12 miles). So there is a lot of room to reach when reaching for the stars! This exercise reintroduces your body to its own reach and your ability to keep reaching farther and farther. But just as you have both lower and higher natures, you need to be grounded in order to fly. So just make sure that you stabilize with your lower as you elevate with the upper. This dynamic will keep you reaching for increasing heights:

1. Stand with your feet hip distance apart. Balance your weight evenly between both feet, which are resting flat on the floor in their natural parallel position.
2. Choose one non-shifting point of focus in front of you.
3. Slightly shift your weight forward on your feet and elevate onto the balls of your feet. Maintain your balance.
4. When you feel ready, raise your arms above your head, as if reaching for the ceiling. Extend through your fingers as if they could grab the stars. If you feel balanced enough, lift your gaze to between your hands. Smile.
5. Feel one energetic force directing your body up and up while, at the same time, another one roots your feet toward the ground.
6. To exit the reach, release your arms by your sides and lower onto flat feet.
7. Practice as many times as you feel comfortable.

If balance is eluding you today, perform this exercise on flat feet. Its most important element is the dynamic of the lift, the grounding of your feet combined with the elevation you feel as your torso and head and hands aspire for great heights. The magic is in the reach itself, not the actual height.

Highest-Self Meditation: To Cultivate Your Higher Nature

Imagine that part of you knows exactly who you are and what you came here to do—you in your wisest, clearest, most elevated capacity. Free from drama, concern, fear, desire, a demanding ego, and with vision into your past, present, future, and the purpose of it all. That is your highest self. Not bad, eh? Whether you realize it or not, you are always connected to this etheric version of yourself. And you always have the choice to make that connection conscious. Give it a try with this meditation, which allows you to access, experience, and learn from your highest nature:

1. Take a comfortable, cross-legged seat on the floor that you are able to maintain for the duration of the meditation. Use cushions for support, if necessary. Turn off your cell phone and set an alarm for ten minutes.
2. Close your eyes and rest your palms, facing up, in your lap.
3. Create an image of yourself in your mind's eye. Just you as you are, no location or other individuals. You can be wearing and doing anything.
4. Feel how that image feels, with honesty and without judgment. Connect with it.
5. Now, create an image of you that represents you at your highest, best, most supreme self. You can look just like you, or an angel, a glowing goddess, a superhero, a centaur. It does not matter what you look like. Allow your imagination to roam free! Be as specific as possible in your depiction: What is the color of your hair? The design of your clothes? What expression is on your face? The more detailed you can be, the better.
6. Feel how that image feels—you will know when you are there. And if you want that image to feel a certain way (for example ecstatic, abundant, compassionate), feel free to imbue it with those feelings.
7. Bring the two images—of your current and highest incarnations—closer together until they merge into one.
8. Rest in this feeling and knowledge of you as your highest self until the alarm sounds.

Ten minutes is simply a starting point. Feel free to start with a longer meditation or increase its length. You should find it a pleasant, heartwarming, and heart-lightening experience.

Practice Discipline: To Tame Your Lower Nature

The Sagittarius British Prime Minister Winston Churchill is popularly credited with saying, "Continuous effort—not strength or intelligence—is the key to unlocking our potential."[1] In other words: practice makes perfect. Practice disciplining your lower nature to allow your higher to shine forth. Harness your weaknesses to develop into strengths, ignorance into knowledge, poverty into abundance, sadness into joy. Self-discipline, like a muscle, can be developed. And it greatly behooves the Centaur nature, which would otherwise happily gallop astray. Start with the following:

1. Schedule two minutes (timed with an alarm) a day for this exercise. Choose a time during the day when you can be alone. Commit to this exact schedule for three weeks.

2. Take a Post-it Note (any color and shape, as long as it stands out from the wall) and post it on the wall at eye level from a seated position. Sit on the opposite side of the room in a comfortable position and focus your gaze and mental attention on the Post-it. Do not think about anything, even that you are looking at a piece of paper. If you lose your focus before the end of the two minutes, that is okay. Return it to the image as soon as you realize it shifted away. The first step in discipline in this exercise is committing to the practice and regularly showing up for it. The disciplining of the mind for two minutes (and beyond) follows.

3. If you are able to focus for the full time on multiple occasions in a row without your concentration drifting, increase the timer to three, then four minutes, and so on.

4. Three weeks is the minimum recommended time frame for pattern change. But feel free to continue for longer and let the practice evolve in a way that works for you.

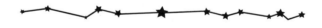

Summary

★ Your hips are the regions related to Sagittarius. These sturdy joints—which move the thighs—have a large range of motion, able to direct you wherever you choose to go.

★ Sagittarius is the ninth sign of the zodiac cycle. Its energy acknowledges your higher and lower natures, and it asks that your higher one lead the show.

★ If your visionary Sagittarius nature becomes either righteous or reckless, your hips might experience different symptoms (e.g., tightness, weakness).

★ Align your inner Sagittarius through questions, exercises, and activities that focus on your hips. Use them to aim for the stars in order to inform your earthly direction.

Note

1. Matthew Radmanesh, *Cracking the Code of Our Physical Universe: The Key to a New World of Enlightenment and Enrichment* (Bloomington, IN: AuthorHouse, 2006), 155.

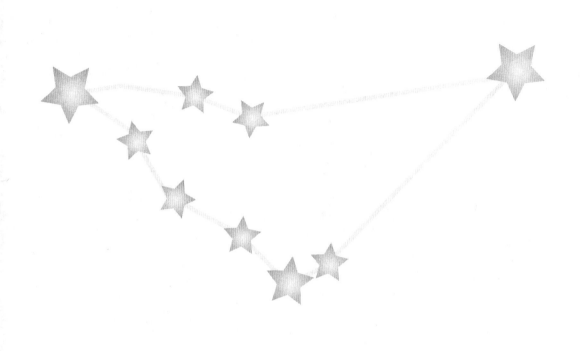

11

Knees of the Seagoat

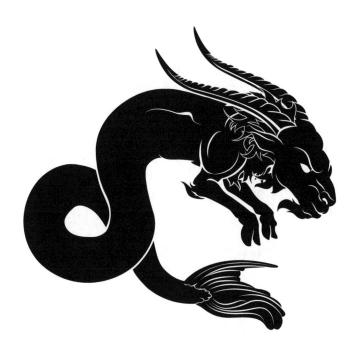

♑ CAPRICORN

Birth date: December 22–January 19
Body region: Knees
Theme: Act Responsibly for
the Greater Good

In the prior sign of Sagittarius, the world is a chalice filled—and ready to be filled—with wisdom. Everything is a teaching, a lesson, an opportunity. Capricorn enters the picture having learned a lot and now ready to distill the knowledge into something useful and practical. Not for herself, necessarily, but for her surrounding community. The Capricorn is the zodiac's realist; here to meet society directly and then do everything she can to take it one step further. She is ambition and willpower incarnate, here to channel these abilities into actions on behalf of the greater good.

Your Body: Knees

Capricorn is an earth sign and as such is stable. Practical. Enduring. Nonetheless, she is still driven forward to accomplish, and it is her knees—the body region related to the sign—that take her there. Her knee joints embody this inner trade-off between stability and mobility, as a region that is required to support the weight of the entire body above, while moving it on the ground below. The design that generates this trade-off is a modified hinge joint (think of a door as an example of a hinge) comprising three different bones (the tibia, femur, and patella). Each joint flexes and extends the knee while permitting a bit of built-in rotation.

Flexion and extension of the knee move your legs, allowing you to walk to work, kick a soccer ball, and climb a mountain. And *how* you engage in these activities will indicate whether or not you will succeed at doing them over the long term. For example, if you are overdoing an activity or doing it with improper alignment, you will injure your knees despite your best intentions. It is how most joint injuries arise: through a combination of overuse and misuse, which results in degeneration. Many times when this occurs, it is due to an excess of mind over matter instead of minding your matter.

Your Capricorn nature—as well as your knees—requires a balance of both. She reminds us to keep our eye on the prize, to do what it takes to achieve it, and simultaneously to be diligent and dutiful about the steps we take on the way there. Her cause is larger than herself, and it requires patience to happen, just like the time and attention that is required to properly perform a headstand or train for a marathon. If, by contrast, you want to get to the end pose or the end of the race at all costs because that is simply what your mind dictates, then woe be your knees, a susceptible part of the Capricorn.

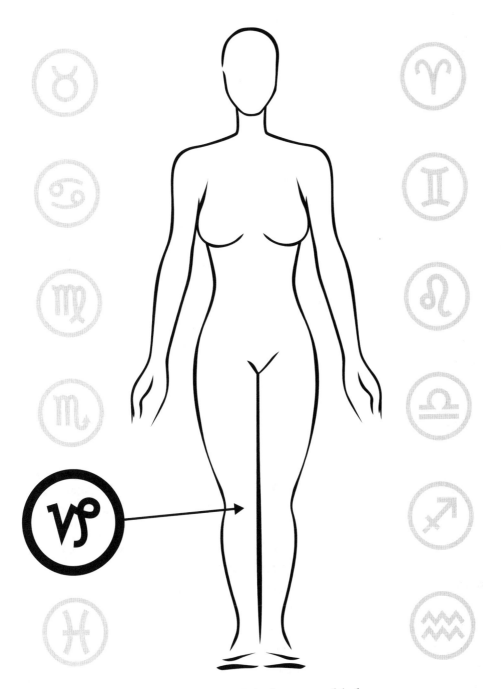

See appendix C for the skeletal structure of the knee.

How do your knees take you where you want to go? Many individuals are not even aware of their knees until something happens to them—until they hurt, ache, or otherwise stop functioning as they are supposed to. And while it is natural that you are more familiar with some parts of your body than others, the knees are good ones to know. So take a moment and reintroduce yourself to this body part that allows you to act in so many ways every day:

1. Sit down and roll your pants up or put on shorts so you can view your knee joints in all their glory. Note that they have curves and contours, as well as fronts, backs, and sides.

2. One joint at a time, use both of your hands to feel the knee. Feel the knee-cap (patella), bony ridges, and surrounding muscles and tendons on all sides. Explore at will, asking yourself questions: What is its temperature (is it cooler or warmer than the surrounding regions)? Do any parts feel tender? Swollen? How does each knee compare to the other? How are they symmetrical and asymmetrical? Sitting as you are now, how do the knees align in relationship to your feet (for example, directed over the second toe, buckling in)?

3. After you feel more familiar with your knees, stand up and walk around. How do your knees naturally move you? With conviction, stability, forward momentum? A limp? Buckling?

For the four-legged land goat, the knees are an integral part of its existence. In fact, some goats suffer from a certain type of viral arthritis that primarily affects the knee joints and are forced to lie down a lot and even walk on their knees to avoid bringing together the joint surfaces. Ultimately, the knee injury might even lead to the goat's demise as it is unable to sustain itself. The mythic Seagoat can help us heed the lessons of her zodiac sign before your knees reach this point! It simply requires your awareness of their existence combined with deliberate action—deliberate steps, runs, and jumps toward your end goal. Imagine if you aimed for and achieved your goals with healthy deliberation. How would your body feel? How about the rest of you? Be the goat walking up the mountain, with each step chosen, calculated, and practical. Be in it for the long run, not easily deterred. With proper time and attention, your outcome will be achieved. Have faith that you will endure.

The Stars: Capricorn

Act Responsibly for the Greater Good

To act is to exert energy or force, and it is in Capricorn's nature to initiate activity. Different from the other signs in the category, though, she acts with the outcome in mind.

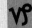

Origin of the Seagoat according to ancient mythology: Pan was the son of Hermes, a god, and Aix, a goat. As such, he was part goat and the goat herder's god. One day in the woods, he had to escape the monster Typhon. He did so by giving himself a fish tail and diving into the water. Later, he helped Zeus in battle with this monster, and as a reward, the king of the gods placed Pan among the stars as the constellation Capricorn.

Think about your daily life and all of your daily actions—they are countless! From brushing your teeth to engaging in a conversation, you do many different things. But how many of those tasks do you undertake with a specific goal in mind? For instance, when you brushed your teeth this morning, did you scrub with the intention to remove plaque from each tooth . . . or did you move through the motions on autopilot, thinking about your upcoming workday? Chances are it was the latter. And that's fine! The point is to recognize that for every time you act, you choose (even unwittingly) a focus—and for our Seagoat nature, it tends to be the outcome. In their worldview, there is simply no need to do something unless it serves some practical purpose. The Seagoat is not here for the journey but for its end goal, like her namesake goat that steadily climbs the mountaintop with the enduring intent to reach its summit.

Just as the four-footed animal makes the ascent as a strong and steadfast climber, the constellation's goat is patient as well. Outcome-based action is a time game, and with her eye on the prize, it does not matter how long it takes Capricorn to get there. She is in it to win it, which, in terms of her zodiac sign and energy, means creating lasting structures that make a mark on the world. Many times, these structures are not physical but theoretical. For instance, Andreas Vesalius, the sixteenth-century Capricorn anatomist, accurately delineated the structure of the human form and compiled his findings in a comprehensive book—making him the founding father of modern human anatomy. About a century later, Sir Isaac Newton—among many superlative scientific achievements—delineated the structure of our physical universe in terms of three laws that describe bodies in motion. Looking even further afield was the astronomer-astrologer-mathematician Johannes Kepler, who helped humanity more realistically structure the cosmos with a telescope that boasted larger fields and higher magnifications.

> ♑ The Capricorns who helped structure our modern-day understanding of science read like a Who's Who list: James Watt (developed horsepower), Louis Braille (developed a reading system for the blind), Louis Pasteur (discovered the principles behind vaccination and pasteurization), Albert Schweitzer (a Nobel Prize–winning medical missionary), and Benjamin Franklin (invented bifocals and the lightning rod).

These scientific Seagoats might not have known, exactly, what the outcomes of their mathematical, physical, and astronomical endeavors were going to be, but they knew that their scientific queries were important and that the answers were likely even more so. So despite the rocky terrain that enabled their immortality today (do not be fooled into thinking that their successes were without failures), they all spent a lifetime climbing. But there is one more piece to the puzzle: In addition to the *what*, there is the *how*. *How* should we act? And the answer for most Capricorns—or any of us when we're engaging our Capricorn energy—is responsibly. For example, Kepler viewed his scientific work as religious duty, a responsibility to understand the workings of a God who created humankind in his image.

You likely feel responsible for a lot of people and things in your life too. Perhaps you feel responsible for your kids' development, your mother's health, your house's upkeep, your duties at work . . . the list goes on and on. This feeling is effectively a sense of obligation that arises from within yourself and extends to others. An accountability for who you are and how you live, inside and out.

When you take ownership of your life, everything starts with you . . . but given that you exist within many greater contexts (family, neighborhood, city, country, world), ownership ultimately extends to the greater whole. Both are related. Which is why taking care of your health—including very personal decisions like how much you eat, sleep, and exercise—affects your contribution at the community level. It is hard to be a productive member of society when you are sick at home! And even though there are many valid reasons for why you got sick—from ill coworkers to undue stress—the responsibility for your health ultimately starts and stops with you, with your choices and decisions. Forget right and wrong (you moved beyond that dichotomy in Gemini). More importantly: Are you making the decisions that are best for you at any given time using what you've got? Are you aware of and willing to accept the trade-offs and compromises? Do you accept that your actions may lead to unforeseen consequences that can be seen as both good *and* bad? That is the essence of acting responsibly.

Acting responsibly is a way of exerting control over your life instead of becoming a victim to it, a way of moving through each day as the master of your own destiny, come hell or high water. And the reward—self-empowerment—is well worth the challenge. Sure, external factors and forces exist that help drive or derail you, but they are not mutually exclusive with your piece of the puzzle. It is like the old adage says: you can lead a horse to water, but you cannot make it drink. Ultimately, and despite all mitigating factors, it is up to the horse, or Seagoat in this case, to drink. The Seagoat's sense of responsibility takes many forms, but a big one includes civic duty—a social force that binds the Capricorn to types of action congruent with that force.

Imagine that you are standing at a crosswalk with no cars coming. You are in a rush, and it would greatly behoove you to cross the street. But if you did—and even if nobody got harmed in the process—you would be breaking the law. A law that was put into place to protect pedestrians at large. To ensure the welfare of not just one hustling walker but of a bustling community of them. How then, do you act? How and when do you choose to uphold your perceived personal good versus the greater one? For Seagoats, the greater good is the driving force. Why act to affect just one individual when you can benefit many? This far into the zodiac cycle, the self is only one piece of a much larger puzzle that makes you *you*. So acting on behalf of others— whether they're your family or surrounding society—is the same thing as achieving your own goals, which means that your inner Seagoat needs to keep others in mind to feel fulfilled.

That said, the Capricorn nature is not devoid of ego identity. We all need a sense of self—for even though we are all but drops of water in the proverbial ocean, we are each our own drop, nonetheless. And our Seagoat knows this well. Although it is the greater force of the ocean that carries her forth, she is acutely aware of the implications for her personally, especially the status she might achieve, whether in her workplace, family, or society. It is the natural reward for her long, arduous ascent up the mountain. To reiterate, though: status should not be the drive but a desired outcome.

> Familiar with the phrase "The ends justify the means"? It paraphrases the philosophy of Niccolò Machiavelli, a Capricorn rising sign instructing a prince on how to achieve and maintain power in *The Prince*. The "prince" he was instructing? Lorenzo de' Medici, a governor of Florence (to whom the book was dedicated) . . . and a fellow Capricorn.

Lessons

The Capricorn Seagoat, like any goat, is a good rock climber. She proceeds in a manner that is stable, enduring, independent, and strong. This Seagoat has work to do, and not much can get in the way of her meticulous plans. This stands true for even her own needs, as the Seagoat is inclined to put her family and work interests before her own. Hence, her association with the greater good.

A cautionary tale of how exclusive status-seeking does not end well for the Capricorn involves Cronus, king of the Titans (a.k.a. Saturn, Capricorn's ruling planet). Against the protestations of his wife, Cronus ate all his children in order to maintain his throne. Until, that is, his son Zeus was born and led an earth-shaking rebellion against his father that ultimately dethroned Cronus and established Zeus as king.

To reliably execute her responsibilities, however, she cannot completely put her needs aside—and neither can you. So it is important that you learn to help your Capricorn nature connect personally to the greater good, not see it as separate. Her needs . . . yours . . . theirs . . . mine . . . all are intertwined. But with such a serious and steadfast nature, the Seagoat can all too readily dismiss her own welfare. If this occurs—if you refuse to tune in to what you want—melancholy will prevail. Most of the time, the Seagoat is willing to forego her emotions to do what she perceives needs to get done. But make no mistake—even though she is typically not considered warm and fuzzy, the Seagoat has many emotions. And if they are not properly acknowledged and channeled, they can manifest as very capricious behavior. So your inner Seagoat typically needs to loosen her reins and have just a bit of fun on her own terms, lest she overdo the doing (to which, of all the joints, the knee joint may fall prey).

Physical manifestations of an obligated Capricorn nature may include:

★ Tight, contracted muscles and tendons surrounding the knee joint (i.e., from the thigh or leg)
★ Achy pain or discomfort in the knee when moving or sitting
★ Restricted or rigid range of motion of the leg
★ Locked knees
★ Crackling or crunching sound heard or sensation felt upon movement
★ Excess fluid around the joint
★ Shin splints

On the other hand, if the Seagoat is too driven by her personal desires—versus those of a greater good—then she might find that her plans are unsupported. That, regardless of her diligent and patient planning and plotting, they are not coming to fruition, even over the long haul. In effect, this is when you feel worn out from a steady drive and progression . . . that's just in the wrong direction. It is akin to over-using your knees, and improperly at that (like running marathons with knees lifting too high).

Physical manifestations of a self-serving Capricorn nature may include:

★ Weak muscles and tendons surrounding the knee joint (i.e., from the thigh or leg)
★ Sensation of weak knees, buckling, or giving out
★ Achy pain or discomfort in the knee when moving or sitting
★ Hyperextension
★ Poor knee alignment

How responsibly do *your* knees move you? Whether they feel obligated, self-serving, or somewhere in between, the key is listening to your body and giving it what it needs. To stretch tight knees or strengthen weak ones, awaken your inner Capricorn with the questions and exercises that follow.

Your Body and the Stars

The following will serve as your personal guide to embodying the Capricorn stars. Use them to act responsibly for the greater good.

Questions

★ How would you characterize the nature of your daily actions (planned, purposeful, flying by the seat of your pants)?
★ What drives these actions (responsibility, success, excitement, fear)? How do your knees move you to act (achingly, tightly, buckling now and then)?
★ List your many duties. Which are primarily on behalf of others? Which are directed toward yourself?
★ When is the last time you externalized responsibility onto another (like blaming a spouse or co-worker)? Looking back, what was the role you played—your responsibility—in the matter?

★ What does *the greater good* mean to you? Who are its members? In what ways do you feel that you act on its behalf? How do you feel when you act on its behalf?

Exercises

Warrior II Pose: To Act with Strength and Deliberation

"It's a dangerous business, Frodo, going out of your door. . . . You step into the Road, and if you don't keep your feet, there is no knowing where you might be swept off to." This line by Frodo (quoting Bilbo Baggins) comes from Capricorn author J. R. R. Tolkien's epic fantasy novel *The Fellowship of the Ring*.[1] In other words: act with intention, purpose. Know what you are doing and why. One of the best ways for anyone—elf, hobbit, or human—to "keep [their] feet" is to deliberately align the knees and legs that place them. When your knees are positioned straight ahead, they help your feet follow suit. Use this yoga pose to deliberately strengthen and align your knees so they can carry you accordingly.

1. Start in a neutral standing position. Elevate your arms to a T position and step your feet apart so that your ankles align under your wrists. Keep your shoulders down, wrists neutral, and fingers extended.
2. Turn your left foot slightly inward (no more than forty-five degrees) and your right foot ninety degrees outward. Look down to ensure that your left and right heels are in line.
3. Bend your right knee to ninety degrees, so that your thigh comes parallel to the floor. Make sure that your kneecap is positioned directly over your ankle and aligned with your second toe. Your entire foot should be flat on the floor with the arch engaged (no portion of your heel or toes should be lifted). Likewise, all points of your left foot should equally touch the ground.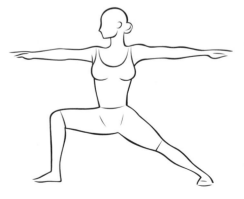
4. Rotate your head to gaze over your right fingertips. Your torso should remain upright, not leaning forward. Stay in this position for five slow and deliberate breaths.

5. Repeat on the other side.

One of the wonders of this pose is that it strengthens the muscles around *both* knees—as long as you properly enter the pose and don't just do it willy-nilly. It strengthens by virtue of engaging a portion of one of the quadriceps femoris muscles known as the vastus medialis oblique (VMO), a group of muscle fibers known for their role in patella tracking and alignment. These fibers are engaged both at the end range of extension (as exemplified by your back knee in the pose) as well as when the knee is bent to a ninety-degree angle and the leg is bearing weight (as exemplified by your front knee). So to reach your desired outcome, make sure that the degree of knee bend is comfortable (not excessive) even if it means you do not reach ninety degrees, and you properly position your knee according to the steps above.

Seated Forward Fold: To Open into Greater Responsibility

Capricorn mystic and poet Khalil Gibran wrote, "Yesterday we obeyed kings and bent our necks before emperors. But today we kneel only to the truth, follow only beauty, and obey only love."[2] What individuals are you responsible to? What greater forces drive your actions? To whom—or what—do you kneel? It is never too late to assess when, where, and how you take responsibility in your daily life. It is never too late to open into new ways of understanding what drives your actions and the realization that, ultimately, it all comes from you. Increase a healthy responsibility with a healthy hamstring stretch for your knees in this seated pose.

1. Sit on the floor with your legs extended straight in front of you. Sit on a cushion if you need help sitting straight atop of your sitting bones. Keep your thighs parallel (not rolling in or out) and legs extended and extend your feet, pushing actively through the heels. Your arms are directly by your sides with the palms pressing into the ground.
2. Keeping your torso long, lean forward from the hip joints (not the waist or back). Bring your chest toward your shins. As you lean forward, hold the

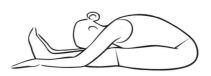

sides of your feet with your hands. If this is not possible, place your hands either on your shins or on the floor beside them.

3. At the extent of your stretch, release your head and neck so that they gently fold forward (your elbows may further bend to help). Remain for ten slow breaths, folding deeper on each exhale.

4. Exit the pose the way you entered, by returning to neutral with a straight torso.

Responsibility does not have to be a burden. It does not have to require tons of effort, and it does not have to hurt. It can be as simple as an acknowledgment that you are the master of your life and all that comes from it. Employ the same ease in this pose. Release the stress and strain, and let the weight of gravity fold you deeper into it.

Knee Circles: To Encompass the Greater Good

As much as life is about you, it turns out that life includes others too. These others surround you whether you like it or not and, in so doing, form different parts of your community. When you act, therefore, your actions do not stand alone. Each action you take is like a pebble thrown into a pond that creates not only its own ring of water but also concentric rings in the surrounding water. In this way, your actions may both intentionally and unintentionally affect others. While outcome is not entirely in your control, you at least have the choice of intention and whether or not it is on behalf of a greater good. Use this exercise to create your own concentric rings through intention-based action.

1. Start in a neutral standing position with feet hip distance apart and hands on your waist.

2. Circle your knees toward the right for five repetitions. Keep your torso upright and not leaning forward. Make sure that the circles are being drawn by your knees, not your hips or shoulders sticking out, and that your feet remain flat on the floor. Maintain the starting distance between your knees as they circle, so they do not bend inward or out.

3. Return to the neutral standing position.

4. Repeat in the other direction.

Shuni Mudra: To Invoke Patience and Discernment

In Kundalini yoga, each finger represents one of the planets and can therefore invoke that planet's energy. The third finger represents Saturn, the ruling planet of Capricorn. Astronomically speaking, Saturn is the sixth planet from the sun. And due to its much larger distance from the sun than Earth (which is the third rock from the sun), it has a much larger orbit. The result: it takes Saturn over 10,800 Earth days to make one orbit around the sun (about thirty times longer than Earth's 365 days). Talk about patience! Saturn is clearly not in a rush. Invoke some patience with a finger mudra that invokes Saturn's enduring energy.

1. Find a comfortable seated position on a chair or on the floor.
2. Place your hands, with palms facing up, on your thighs.
3. On each hand, touch the thumb to the middle finger. Keep the other fingers in a relaxed extension.
4. Close your eyes and connect with the greater wisdom you seek to elicit. Relax and breathe.

This mudra can be performed at any time, for as long as you like.

Take a Bath: To Trust the Outcome

It can be hard to be patient in our society because we are groomed to act. To do do do! And when nothing is visibly happening, it seems as if nothing is happening. But that is typically not the case. Once a wheel is in motion, it is in motion whether you see it or not. Sometimes you just need to wait for it to roll to you; you cannot always be the one rolling it. Trust that you played your part in the process and have faith that what you set in motion will happen in its own time . . . which is often better timing than your mind's. So take some time to take a bath, knowing that even though you are "not doing anything" the bath is doing unto you by allowing the salt to relax the muscles surrounding your knee joints (and the rest of your body as well). All that is required is for you to draw the bath—and then let the bath do the rest.

1. Draw a bath with warm water to your liking.
2. Feel free to create whatever environment will allow you to relax and not worry about the time (such as candlelight). Turn off your phone and any

    other electronics that may call your attention. Setting an alarm for twelve to fifteen minutes will allow you to relax and not regard the time.

3. Place two cups of Epsom salts in the tub and allow a few minutes for the salt to dissolve.
4. Enter the tub and relax until the alarm sounds. Do not use soap in the bath, as it will interfere with the action of the salts.
5. Take up to three Epsom baths weekly.

    Epsom salts, named for a spring in Epsom, England, is not actually salt but a naturally occurring compound of magnesium and sulfate. It has been used as a traditional remedy for a number of ailments, including stress, soreness, muscle tension, and inflammation.

Climb a Mountain: To Remember Your Community

Community can mean any number of things. According to one dictionary, it is a social group of any ilk or size (such as religious, business, or regional). Or it can refer to the locality inhabited by such a group. How do you define your community? Chances are you have many of them, with many intersecting. Check them out by being the Seagoat you are and climbing to the top of whatever mountain, hill, or tall building affords you a view. Look out over your communities—there they are! Whatever hustle and bustle you see around and below encompasses all the different groups to which you belong. The ones that ask you to act responsibly on their behalf, and the ones that give you the support (physical, mental, or emotional) to do so. So go and use your knees to climb up and literally see on whose behalf you are acting and why.

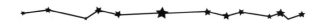

Summary

★ Your knees are the regions related to Capricorn. A balance between stability and mobility, these joints move you wherever—and however—you've chosen to go.

★ Capricorn is the tenth sign of the zodiac cycle. Its energy acknowledges your sense of responsibility and how you employ it patiently and persistently for the greater good.

★ If your practical Capricorn nature dives too deep into work or works for no cause except its own, your knees might experience different symptoms (e.g., pain, locking, crunching).

★ Cultivate your inner Capricorn through questions, exercises, and activities that focus on your knees. Use them to make it to the top of your mountain, making sure to have fun en route.

Notes

1. J. R. R. Tolkien, *The Lord of the Rings: The Fellowship of the Ring* (Boston: Houghton Mifflin, 1965), 83.

2. Khalil Gibran, *The Vision: Reflections on the Way of the Soul* (Ashland, OR: White Cloud Press, 1994), 32.

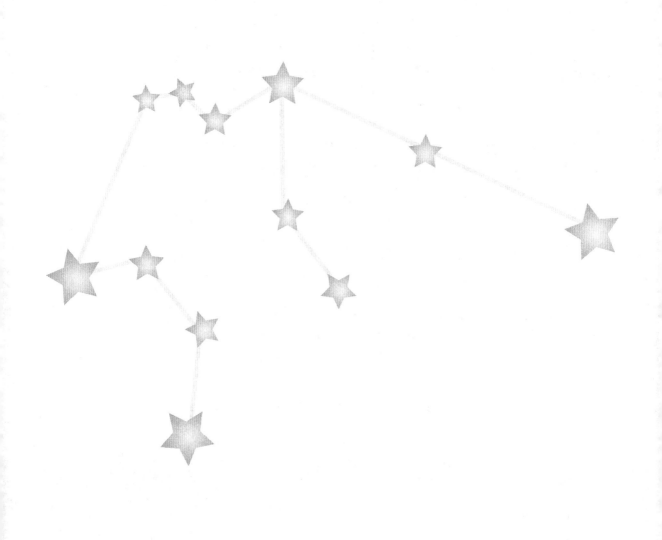

12

Ankles of the Water Bearer

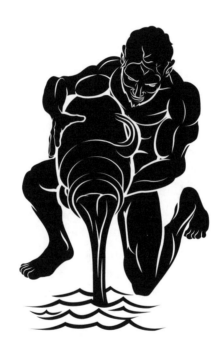

♒ AQUARIUS

Birth date: January 20–February 18
Body region: Ankles
Theme: Awaken the Potential
of a New Age

Now that we have a solid structure for society built by the Capricorn Seagoat, the Aquarian Water Bearer is here to dismantle it! Aquarius is the consummate egalitarian, here to break down Capricorn's hierarchy for what he perceives to be a needed paradigm shift. A new way to meet the collective need with the emphasis on collective. In other words: The Water Bearer is the zodiac's Robin Hood. He is here to awaken the same spirit he sees in himself in all others, ushering in a new age ripe with egalitarian potential.

Your Body: Ankles

Perhaps there is no other part of the body that is as individuated as your ankles, the region of the body related to the Aquarius zodiac sign. While each ankle is primarily able to flex and extend the foot, it is nonetheless the part of your body that determines how you place your foot on the ground (see chapter 13: "Feet of the Fish"). Think about climbing up a rocky hill barefoot and you will understand the importance and nuance involved in your ankle directing your foot—one slight misstep and it is easy to fall!

Composed of only three bones (the tibia and fibula of the leg, and the talus of the foot), the ankle is the region just above your foot—the foot being the only part that actually touches the ground when a bipedal person stands, walks, and moves around. So the movement of your ankle needs to be deliberate because, in placing the foot below, it is also placing the five to six feet of *you* that comes on top. In other words, this humble hinge joint helps determine the refined, individual way you stand and move upon the earth. It transitions the larger movements from the hips and knees above, to the more specific fine-tuning of your feet below, even when you stand (notice that in a prolonged standing position your ankles and feet are never truly still).

Many cultures throughout time have understood that your ankles are more than just bony prominences. In ancient Egypt the ankles were considered areas to be adorned. For this reason, both men and women wore tunics short enough to show off their anklets made of gold, silver, and iron and beads made out of semiprecious stones like amethyst. In India these ankle bracelets were also worn by women for fashion (*payal*) and sometimes symbolized tribal adherence. In the ancient Middle East, two anklets (one on each ankle) might be chained together to produce a clinking sound to both attract attention and shorten the gait, which was considered graceful

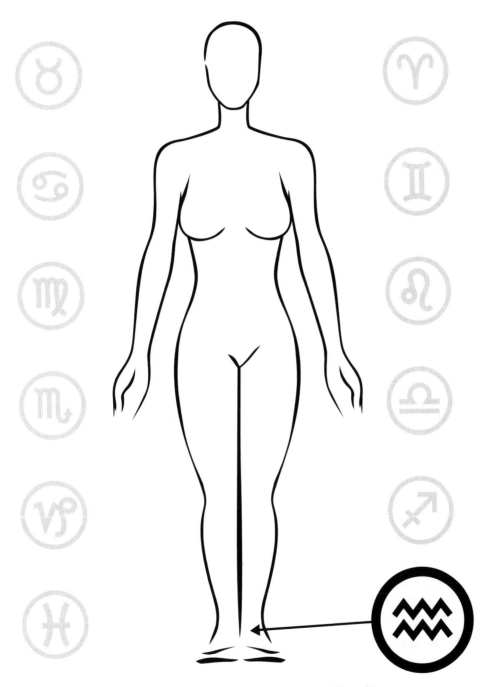

See appendix C for the skeletal structure of the ankle.

and feminine. Some cultures ascribed meaning—like relationship status—to the left versus the right sides. Others, like Victorian England and conservative Islamic states, hid the ankles altogether for reasons of modesty.

When is the last time you looked at *your* ankles, let alone adorned them? These oft-neglected regions say so much about how you do what you do. For instance, how do you stand—with weak, buckling ankles or with stable ones? And what are you standing for? To get on the bus or for your right to sit on it?

 Yup, Rosa Parks—the first lady of civil rights who refused to give up her seat on a bus because of her race—was an Aquarius. As was Abraham Lincoln, who ushered in the first era of American civil rights about a century earlier.

Try this simple stance to start noticing your ankles:

1. Take a standing position with feet hip distance apart.
2. Without moving any part of your body but your neck and head, look down and check out your ankles.
3. Is each sitting bone directly under the knee and above the heels? Or is one or both rolled inward or outward compared to the foot? Just observe.
4. Shift your weight onto your right foot and lift your left foot a few inches off the ground (hold on to a nearby table or chair if needed). What changes occurred in your right ankle? Again, observe.
5. Reverse sides.

That's it. A simple exercise to begin connecting with a seemingly simple joint. But as you shifted onto one foot, you probably felt the ankle's greater complexity, helping you find and maintain your stance. Yet most individuals do not regularly pay attention to this aspect of their individuality—to the particular way in which they walk and stand. And so ankle sprains are one of the most common injuries seen in primary care offices nationwide. Our attention is not focused on our own present and how we are moving through it, as it is often easier to just go with the crowd. If you are following others too much, however, your stance will not be your own and you are more likely to misstep. Every Aquarius needs to take his own stand—it is as important for him as it is for everyone else!

The Stars: Aquarius

Awaken the Potential of a New Age

Each morning you are roused from sleep. Maybe by the light shining through the curtains, an alarm clock, your partner's wakefulness—it does not really matter how since the result is the same: you are awakened. You have been stirred from your slumber or, figuratively speaking, from a state of darkness. You have entered a new day whether it is just a new date on the calendar or a new period in your life, ushering in a new perspective, new ideas, new understandings.

Whatever the case, to be awakened connotes a new, enhanced state of cognizance, one different—and somehow deeper—than you possessed before. When you are awakened, you see a greater truth to any given situation. For instance, you might be awakened to the reality that the story of our healthcare system is different than the actual practice of it. You might be awakened to the fact that your friend—for all of his best intentions—is saying one thing but doing another. You might awaken to the idea that your mind is creating a reality for you that you can choose to change at any moment, which is why you are crying at a movie while the person seated next to you is laughing. There is no end to the many times and ways in which you may be awakened.

The Water Bearer spends his life awakening to his individuality at deeper and deeper levels, like an onion peeled to reveal its many layers. Ultimately, he realizes that his seemingly unique wants and needs actually represent those of the greater whole—that the anger he feels represents an anger that is felt at large (albeit differently by different individuals). So is his hunger. So is his desire to live up to his highest and happiest potential. And so on and so forth.

In physics, potential energy is the energy stored by virtue of position. Like the potential energy of an arrow that is pulled tightly back into the bow just before it is

Another place that rain and potential meet? With Aquarian science fiction writer Jules Verne, who presciently understood that water's components—hydrogen and oxygen—could create fuel. A new idea for his time, and one that is still being explored today.

shot. Or the potential energy of rain before it falls, is processed through a turbine, and ultimately becomes hydroelectric power. Rain is chock-full of potential, not just as a source of electric energy but also as a grower of crops, washer of clothes, cleaner of debris, hydrator of humans, along with potentially being a cause of flooding or, in its absence, drought. So many prospects held in such little drops of H_2O! Which is why the Aquarian constellation is a vessel of water being poured by a man. Throughout many ancient cultures, rain portends possibility of every ilk—from floods to food for soil—a hallmark of the Aquarius sign.

Like water, we all have potential, too, which means that, for all of the qualities you already possess, you can express even more. More love, more creativity, more joy, more success. And while your personal combination of qualities will be different than your mother's, your father's, and the guy's next door, at the meta level you share many of these qualities in common, like love, creativity, joy, and success. So when you wake up to your potential *and* take the next step to act upon it—perhaps through a meditation practice to enhance your inner love, or in an art class to augment your creativity, or by speaking up at work to further your bright ideas—you tacitly give permission to others around you to do the same. Oftentimes it can be challenging to foster your own—let alone another's—potential. But when you do, you make it okay for others to get out there and walk to the beat of their own drum.

There's always the choice: once you become aware of your potential, you decide whether or not to use it. Sure, you can shy away from your own greatness, your own expansion of power. You can keep toeing the main line. But that is not what the Water Bearer part of you is here to do. Your inner Water Bearer is here to live his quirks to the hilt and inspire others to do the same in his inimitably unique way, which may even be original and inventive enough to define a whole new age.

"This is the dawning of"—everyone, sing along—"the age of Aquarius."[1] More than just a famous phrase from the 1970s song named for the zodiac sign, the age is both astronomical and astrological reality. Astronomically speaking, there is no age per se, but there is a shift in the sun's position that occurs every 2,160 or so years, around the spring equinox, when it enters a new zodiac constellation (in this case, into Aquarius from Pisces). Within the world of astrology, this positional shift occurs *and* thereby ushers in the energies of the new sign, which creates an age.

While the official shift into the age of Aquarius is still under discussion (some astrologers posit that it began as early as the 1960s, while others have their eyes on 3600), all agree that the age is happening. Regardless, the Water Bearer energy is not one to wait for a new age to usher itself in. It creates its own ages within ages, so to speak; new paradigms of thought that shift community by influencing how we think, feel, and do. The health of this sign, therefore, requires total and independent freedom to express whatever he is here to do.

Take, for instance Thomas Edison and Charles Darwin—a couple of Aquarians who developed new paradigms of thought during their own historical periods. In 1880, Edison patented the lightbulb and then formed a company to deliver its electricity throughout the country, known today as the General Electric Corporation. Bringing electricity to power society's lights was extremely important; otherwise, you might be reading this book by candlelight instead of on your computer, tablet, or phone. A few decades before, Charles Darwin transformed the way the world thought about the natural world by introducing the concept of natural selection under the umbrella of evolution.

> Aquarian innovators come in all shapes and sizes. A list of female artists, for example, includes Betty Friedan (feminist writer), Ayn Rand (writer and founder of objectivism), Ruth St. Denis (modern dance pioneer), and Gypsy Rose Lee (writer, actress, burlesque performer).

In short: The Water Bearer will always live his own age of Aquarius. It is what he is here for—to awaken to greater realities of man and universe and to bring this understanding to life for the good of all, whether the lightbulb, telescope, or theory of evolution. In this way, he lives his fullest potential while harnessing society's, ushering in the next new age in both regards.

Lessons

Even Aquarius's ruling planet—Uranus—does things its own way. For instance, its tilt is so extreme that, unlike the other planets, it essentially orbits the sun on its side. And unlike the classical planets, which have been viewed since antiquity with the naked eye, Uranus was the first planet to be discovered (albeit accidentally) via telescope by an astronomer in 1781.

Uranus's discovery coincided with the culmination of the age of Enlightenment, an era that heralded—surprise, surprise—individual rights over societal tradition. Beginning in the late 1600s in Europe, the age's movement was to reform society's aristocratic social and political norms, and it led to the rise of the American and French Revolutions, along with a period of literary and artistic Romanticism.

Individual rights, freedom, expression—while concepts in and of themselves—ultimately took shape through men and women who possessed brilliant, original, and liberating perspectives for their times. Yet Aquarius accesses energy and ideals that are not necessarily his. Instead, when you get in touch with your inner Aquarius, you are effectively tapping into an idea whose time has come and acting as the one to bring it to fruition on behalf of your society in your particular manner. It is therefore important that you tune in to your own Aquarian brand of thought and not get lost in all the great thoughts out there. The sea of potential is vast and potentially all consuming. And if you find yourself consumed—unsure of what your thoughts and ideas are versus those of others—you may find yourself grasping at straws as you try to self-define, jumping from one thought form to the next in hopes of securing an identity. In this scenario, you might act radically or lack personal stability. Your challenge, then, is to be secure in your individuality in the face of seemingly infinite potentiality.

Physical manifestations of a radical Aquarius nature may include:

★ Sensation of weakness
★ Hypermobility
★ Swelling
★ Crackling feeling or sound under the skin
★ Snapping sensation
★ Instability
★ Frequent inversion of foot when walking (foot rolls under ankle, with sole pointing inward)

Despite his water vessel, the Water Bearer is a fixed sign, which means that this energy can staunchly and stubbornly stand for something just for the sake of it. This scenario may lead him wayward, in a direction that is not truly his. Or it might make him a committed rebel without a real cause. So it is important that your inner Water Bearer not become rigid in his beliefs. He—and you along with him—needs to go with the flow of the water pouring forth from his vessel—the flow of his ideas, the flow of the times. Otherwise he will become the very establishment he is working against! So your inner Aquarius needs to be firm yet flexible, making sure not to step on other people's toes (and ideals) in the process. Your challenge, then, is to balance the need for individuation with the existing fabric of society. For just as you have individual rights to opine, so do all others.

Physical manifestations of a rigid Aquarius nature may include:

★ Tight, contracted calf muscles
★ Pain, swelling

★ Stiffness in the joint
★ Cramping or charley horse
★ Restricted range of motion, especially visible upon circular rotations
★ A cracking sound or sensation upon movement

How well do your ankles stand your ground? Whether they feel radical, rigid, or somewhere in between, the key is listening to your body and giving it what it needs. To stretch tight ankle muscles or strengthen weak ones, awaken your inner Aquarius with the questions and exercises that follow.

Your Body and the Stars

The following will serve as your personal guide to embodying the Aquarius stars. Use them to awaken the potential of a new age.

Questions

★ What have you recently learned or experienced that awakened you to a new aspect of yourself? Of the world at large?
★ Looking forward, do you see your life as one filled with potential or more of a foregone conclusion? What would need to happen for you to feel full of potential?
★ What new hobbies, classes, or interests have you recently pursued? What did you learn from them? What would you like to learn next?
★ What was your most recent great idea or innovation? Have you ever had a great idea but kept it to yourself for fear of ridicule or worse?
★ How well do your ankles allow you to stand—and move your feet upon—your ground?

Exercises

Tree Pose: To Refine and Strengthen Your Stance
Trees stand tall—up to hundreds of feet, in fact. Yet despite their height, each is endowed with great stability: the ability to retain their stance in storms or gales while rising high. A network of features enables their staunch stance, from a rigid and tapered trunk

to flexible branches, spiraled fibers, and a root system that acts as the tree's anchor. Your anchors—your body's roots—are the feet that you plant onto the ground and the ankles that place and move them while there. Use this tree pose to feel how *you* connect to the ground. Feel how dynamic your stance is, how you have the power to keep refining it, and how you become stronger in the process!

1. Stand in a neutral position with your feet hip distance apart. Shift your weight onto your right leg.
2. Bend your left knee to lift your left foot. Place the sole of your left foot on the inside of your right thigh (using your hands if necessary). Your left toes should be pointing down toward the ground.
3. Press your hands together in a prayer position in front of your chest (the more advanced may raise their arms into "branches" overhead, and lift the gaze accordingly). Or, if you need help with balance, hold on to a table or chair.
4. Engage your core. For further stability, press the sole of your left foot into your standing thigh and your thigh back into your foot.
5. Find a focus directly in front of you and maintain it, and the position, for five breaths.
6. Once you are comfortably balanced, feel how your foot moves side to side and back and forth upon the floor. Then, shift your mental focus to your ankle and notice how the ankle moves in response to the forces from both the ground and the foot . . . as well as directs them. Now, intentionally, stabilize your ankle to minimize its movements and those of the foot; this is one way of exerting your power to refine your own stance.
7. Repeat on the other side.

If the full tree position challenges your balance, modify it by placing your foot on your calf or ankle; your toes may even touch the floor. (Just be sure not to put your foot on the inside of the knee, to avoid injury.) Finding a strong and balanced stance is the most important focus of this exercise—not foot height.

Ankle Circles: To Awaken

Who knew awakening was as simple as circling your ankles? Well, awakening may take any number of forms, big or small. And sometimes the greatest gifts are in the most surprising packages . . . not the ones your mind was necessarily expecting or hoping for. Use this exercise to awaken to your ankles—likely a part of your body you have not spent much time intentionally exploring. All of your physical bits and pieces hold wisdom—something new to learn and understand about yourself—and your ankles are no different. Rather than just following the rest of your body throughout the day, take some weight off this unfamiliar region and allow your ankles to move as they are meant to, through their natural range of motion with joint-opening circles.

1. Sit comfortably in a chair with your back straight, shoulders open and relaxed, and chin parallel to the ground. Your feet should be uncrossed, with feet flat on the floor. If possible, do this barefoot.
2. Keeping your left foot flat on the floor, lift your right leg and circle your right ankle clockwise for ten slow counts. Spread your toes (even within your shoes). Gently place your foot back on the ground.
3. Reverse directions and circle counterclockwise.
4. Repeat on the left side.

Toe Stand: To Cultivate Your Potential

Now that you have reconnected to and awakened your ankles with the aforementioned circles, this exercise will help your ankles do what they—and you—were meant to do. In other words: flex and extend your feet. These are simple movements with much potential that, chances are, you have yet to access. Just ask any ballerina who spent six years practicing standing on her toes to one day don "toe" shoes and stand *en pointe* (on the tops of her toes)! She had to create a foundation to be able to open to a larger world of opportunity—like performing as the soloist in *Swan Lake*.

1. Walk around barefoot for a few minutes to make sure that your calf muscles, which move the ankle, are limber and ready to move safely.
2. Stand with your feet hip distance apart and your weight evenly distributed between both feet. Make sure that your feet are in their natural parallel position and toes are spread as evenly and widely as possible.
3. Spread your arms into a T.
4. Gently bend both of your knees.
5. Raise both of your heels off of the ground, keeping the balls of the feet on the floor. Your entire body should subsequently raise as one unit.
6. Inhale, engage your core, and straighten your knees.
7. Exhale and—maintaining straight knees and an engaged core—lower your heels to the floor. Keep your arms elevated.
8. Repeat for five inhale-exhale cycles.

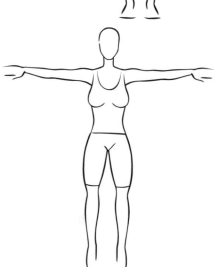

Every day presents new possibilities—including those concerning your balance. If you are feeling more balanced, hold the last *relevé* for as long as possible before descending in a controlled manner. If you are feeling less balanced, perform the entire exercise holding on to a table or chair in front of you; stand as close to the object as needed to maintain as straight as possible torso.

Squat: To Strengthen Your Stance

Once upon a time, before you stood, you squatted. You did it as a baby, and babies have done it collectively for likely the couple hundred thousand years of our evolutionary history. In a way, a squat is preparation for standing, allowing a baby to sense the ground with both feet (in a bipedal stance) while preserving the functional utility of his hands. It is also grounding, as it requires a firm stance to not only squat down but also return to a standing position using nothing but strength and balance.

Chances are, however, that despite your early training, squats rarely make it into your daily routine (unless you live in some indigenous cultures where squats are naturally employed hundreds of times a day). Nowadays, your seat is likely a couch or chair. So dust off the cobwebs and re-find your squat! It will help strengthen your stance.

1. Stand with your feet slightly wider than shoulder distance apart (approximately the width of a generic exercise mat). Both feet are flat on the floor. Slightly angle your feet outward. Place your hands on your waist.
2. Gently and deeply bend your knees and hips, lowering yourself into a squatted position. Your torso might lean forward.
3. When you have reached the extent of your bend, place your hands in a prayer position in front of your chest, with the elbows inside of the knees, gently pressing the knees outward to come over the second toe. This should help the buttocks come closer toward the feet.
4. Use the leverage of your elbows against your knees to help strengthen and lengthen your torso.
5. Hold the position for five breaths.
6. Straighten your knees and hips to return to standing. You may keep your arms in prayer position. Try to stand up with as few extraneous movements as possible.
7. Repeat two more squats (moving your hands to your waist, if necessary, to facilitate the descent).
8. After exiting the final squat and returning to standing, release your arms to the sides. Shake your body out.

If your Achilles tendons are tight and prevent you from descending into the pose, place a rolled-up mat or blanket under your heels. If you have any knee or hip injuries, flex the affected joint(s) within a pain-free range of motion, and hold for only as long as is comfortable; one round sitting atop a block may even be enough.

Achilles' heel is a nickname for your calcaneal tendon. It comes from Greek mythology, in which the demigod Achilles—as a baby—is dipped into the River Styx in order to gain immortality. His mother holds him by his heel so all of her son's body derives the river's benefits—except his heel, of course, which is left out. Years later, in the Trojan War, Achilles is killed by an arrow shot into the one place he is mortal and therefore vulnerable—his Achilles' heel.

Mantra: To Usher in a New Age

Om is probably the most famous of the Sanskrit mantras, frequently used in yoga classes at the beginning or end or both. Sound is a form of vibration, and the sound *om* represents the vibration of the universe, the underlying frequency at which all form was created and is maintained. It represents both the manifest and unmanifest and, when chanted, it harmonizes your individual resonance with the resonance of the universe. In other words, it cultivates the universal through the individual. It helps you get in touch with your inner god. What does your inner divinity have in store for you? And for your contributions to the world? You won't know until you open the door to a whole new world and find out.

> Does a connection between sound and divinity sound familiar? The opening verse of the Gospel of John in the King James Version of the Bible reads, "In the beginning was the Word, and the Word was with God, and the Word was God."

1. Choose a space and time that is free from interruption.
2. Find a comfortable seat on the floor, sitting cross-legged upon a cushion, pillow, or block if needed (if cross-legged is not possible, find an easeful position sitting upright on the floor; if this position is not possible, sit on a chair).
3. Rest your hands in your lap, palms facing up. Gently close your eyes.
4. Feeling the vibration originate in your chest, produce the sound *om* (pronouncing it as the *o* in *yoke*). Allow the sound to be long and expansive as it rises. Feel the vibration all the way from your chest, up through your throat, and as it leaves your lips.
5. Repeat two more times.
6. Remain seated with eyes closed and feel the residual vibration throughout your body before getting up.

For greatest effect, practice the mantra daily. The inherently innovative Aquarians tend to get bored by routine, so do not worry about picking a specific time—do it when the moment suits you.

Get to Class: For Innovation and Variation

What floats *your* fancy? Sculpture? Dance? Math? English lit? Kick up your daily routine by taking a class that adds a different experience. Aquarian energy likes to be introduced to a variety of activities. Plus, a group setting ensures that you get out of your laboratory (which might even be just in your head) and into the world . . . the one you are primed to shift. Without even trying, you pick up on other people's energies, keeping what suits you and discarding the rest. It is how the Water Bearer takes in a variety of new perspectives in order to create his own unique blend.

Summary

★ Your ankles are the regions related to Aquarius. These complex joints allow you to refine and stand your ground in your unique way.
★ Aquarius is the eleventh sign of the zodiac cycle. Its energy acknowledges your idealistic and innovative potential, which allows you to tap new perspectives in order to usher in a new age.
★ If your rebellious Aquarius nature swings to either the rigid or the radical, your ankles might experience different symptoms (e.g., swelling, crackling).
★ Access your inner Aquarius through questions, exercises, and activities that focus on your ankles. Use them to help you stand for what you believe is right—a fair and free future for all.

Note
1. The Fifth Dimension, "Aquarius/Let the Sunshine In (The Flesh Failures)," by James Rado and Gerome Ragni (lyrics) and Galt MacDermot (music), on *The Age of Aquarius* (Los Angeles, CA: Liberty Records), 1969.

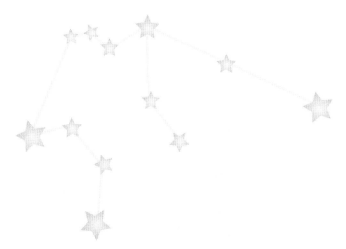

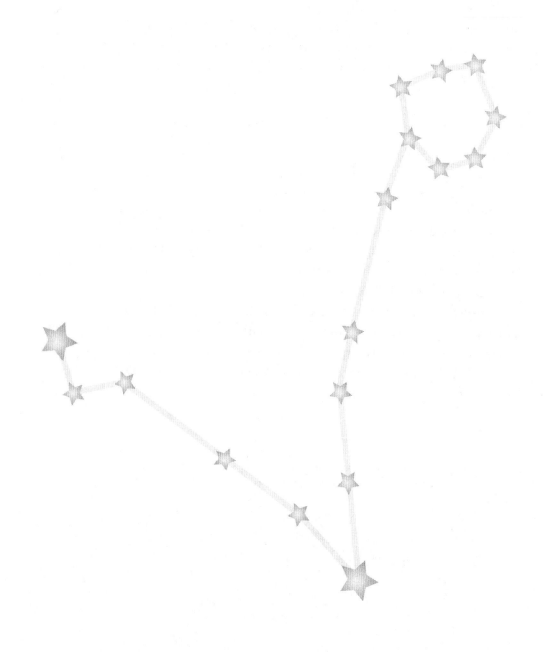

13

Feet of the Fish

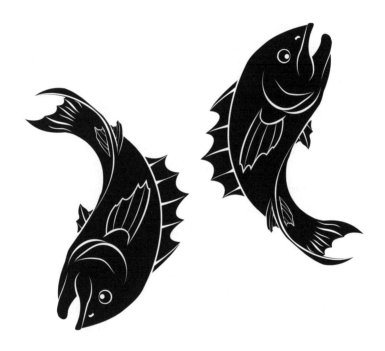

♓ PISCES

Birth date: February 19–March 20
Body region: Feet
Theme: Integrate Spirit into Matter

With Pisces, the zodiac comes full cycle. The eleven preceding signs have been lived and learned, and now it is up to Pisces to take their wisdom and apply it, to ground their cosmic teachings here on Earth. The Fish, therefore, is divinity in the flesh. She holds the spirit of Aries all the way through Aquarius. And her form is just as important as her spirit! For, just like water cannot serve its purpose until it is poured into an appropriate container, neither can the flowing spirit of the Pisces. She needs a vessel, a physical conduit to bring the starry lessons of the zodiac to life. And so, just like the vesica pisces—embodied in her constellation's symbol of two fish swimming in opposite directions—she is here to merge two seeming opposites, spirit and matter, and remind us that they are one.

♓ Over time, the *vesica pisces*—classically, a depiction of two circles of the same radius intersecting—has represented everything from fish, to Jesus, to a solar eclipse, to a geometric matrix used to design ancient religious buildings.

Your Body: Feet

Each foot—the body region related to the Pisces sign—is a marvel of Mother Nature that contains almost thirty bones, over twenty joints, and eleven sets of intrinsic muscles (in contrast, the much larger region of the thigh, which has a similar number of muscles, has only one bone and two joint articulations). Working together, your feet form the weight-bearing platform on which you stand upright, a defining feature of the human species. From that platform, your feet propel you forward and backward, sensing the earth as you go—walking, jogging, and yoga-ing as you see (and become) fit. In fact, your feet possess some of the most sensitive skin in your whole body specifically for that reason—to sense how to best connect you to the ground below. (Don't be fooled by rough corns and calluses! These thickenings of skin form to protect the sensitive skin beneath.)

As the connection between all of you and the earth, your feet play a very important role in your life. They are grounding not just your anatomical and physiological bits and pieces but also all of the visions, dreams, fears, hopes, and love that dwell inside. Besides, how else would you get to your beloved Tuesday yoga class? Even if you take the bus, it is your feet that are walking you on board.

Despite its extensive utility, however, the modern-day foot is no stranger to neglect. While intended for barefoot running through the sand dunes of Namibia, it is, instead, strapped into a three-inch heel on the cement sidewalks of New York City. The unnatural arrangement of the foot required for placement in such a shoe results

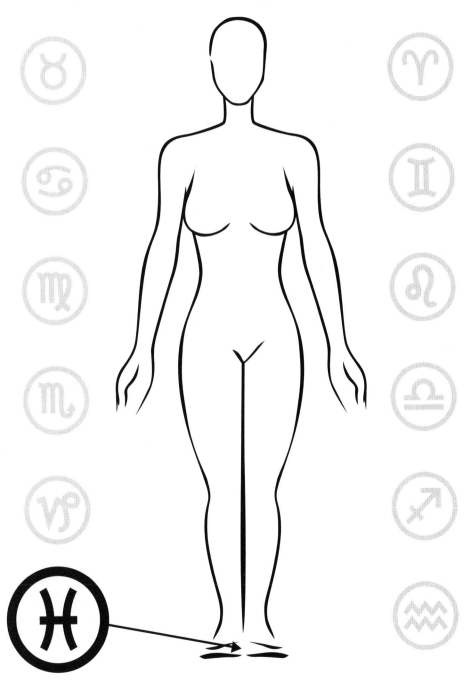

See appendix C for the skeletal structure of the foot.

not only in foot abuse but also in a misappropriation of the entire body's structure. High heels overtire foot, leg, and thigh muscles that would otherwise remain inactive; they stretch and strain ligaments that are not prepared to endure constant presssure; they tax the joints of the ankle and foot, and impinge upon important vessels and nerves.

High heels, however, are just one example: socks, shoes, chairs, pavement, modern transportation, and always having somewhere to go all remove you from the ground. Indeed, if you are the average American, it's likely been a while since you have stood barefoot, two feet planted firmly on natural ground, present in your body for a full five minutes. In removing you from *the* ground, all of these modern accoutrements remove you from your *personal* ground—the way that you were meant to be and operate, free from external interference.

Why is grounding so important? Because it is how you take both the tangible and the intangible parts of you and live them on this planet. This is a big deal for the otherwise free-spirited Pisces energy that would float happily in the clouds. But Earth is made of more than clouds and our society would not benefit if all of the Fish's hard-learned lessons stayed in your head instead of becoming manifest in words, interactions, art, fashion, and other modalities that could inspire more rather than the few.

So you need to connect to your feet in order to connect your Pisces nature to her ground, to the matter that will make her spirit accessible to the physical world. How grounded do you feel on your own two feet? Try this to see:

1. Wear shoes and socks (or high heels) that remove you from the floor.
2. Stand upright with feet hip distance apart, arms elongated by your sides. Weight should be evenly balanced between both feet.
3. Close your eyes and gently shift your weight back and forth, left and right, and sense your connection to the floor below.
4. Return to your neutral stance and open your eyes.
5. Take off your shoes and socks so that you are barefoot. Shake out your feet.
6. Stand upright with feet hip distance apart, arms elongated by your sides. Weight should be evenly balanced between both feet.
7. Close your eyes and gently shift your weight back and forth, left and right, and sense your connection to the floor below.
8. Return to standing and open your eyes, noticing the difference between standing with shoes on and without.

For some of you, standing barefoot might have felt a bit jarring, as you are not used to the full and sensitive extent of your connection with the ground. You are used to being "protected" in foot armor. For others, standing barefoot might have been liberating. It might have felt like a breath of air finally allowing you to release into and connect with parts of yourself that had been kept artificially contained. For all, barefoot is how you and your body were evolutionarily designed to be. And in a society that removes you from your natural substrate, it is never too late to reintroduce yourself to your feet, becoming increasingly aware of how they feel as parts of your body and appreciating their special role in your life. (Read chapter 4: "Hands of the Twins" to review the parallel structures of the hands and feet. Sure, the feet lack opposable big toes, but with a similar intricacy of bones and joints, they are amenable to a similar slew of fine movements . . . which is why cultures that let their feet be feet, like in Southeast Asia, are even able to use them to sew!)

The Stars: Pisces

Integrate Spirit into Matter

Integration is a synthesis, a union, an incorporation of seemingly separate parts into a greater whole. Just like how a hundred puzzle pieces coalesce into a larger picture of a beach or horse, or how blending some flour, salt, and yeast—with the help of an oven—makes bread. Integration, of course, is not just physical; you might combine various thoughts and references from a semester's worth of English class into a new thesis. Or you might have enough positive experiences with and feelings toward one individual that, over time, she becomes someone you consider a friend.

These examples demonstrate physical, mental, and emotional constructs that you regularly integrate into your daily life. Pisces, however, goes one step further and introduces spirit into the equation so that everyone is a walking, talking integration of body, emotions, mind, *and* spirit. For instance, take any given interaction with love: you likely use your mind to think about love (what it means to you), access your emotions in order to feel it (the warming of your heart each time you see a loved one), use your arms to physically express it (giving hugs), and tap into your spirit to detect love in its many forms (you see it shining bright in your canine companion's eyes). Without one of these elements—body, emotions, mind, spirit—your personal experience of love would fall short. Which is why most individuals spend their lives seeking to authentically express their entire selves—from matter to spirit—even if they are not quite sure what that looks like, or even what it means.

One of history's most iconic depictions of spirit meeting the mundane appears on the ceiling of the Vatican's Sistine Chapel, by the renowned Pisces artist Michelangelo. At the material level, Michelangelo did not do much more than mix, blend, and otherwise integrate a series of oil colors and forms together. But by breathing life into Genesis's opening passages with his depiction of man and God reaching out to connect, he also integrated spirit. Which made all the difference in the world! Suddenly, a few brushstrokes became more than just wall (or, rather, ceiling) art and, instead, a timeless emblem of dust being brought to life by the spirit of God . . . a job so well rendered that millions of men and women visit it every year.

When spirit and matter become one, duality no longer exists. You may recall this theme emerging earlier in the zodiac with the Gemini Twins. There, you were introduced to two sides of the human coin—more or less corresponding to the innate duality of our nature. With Pisces, these elements are now integrated, with man living as spirit and spirit taking life as man—different expressions of the same thing. Pisces thereby heralds the end of duality by allowing the etheric, nebulous world of spirit to no longer be considered separate but, rather, part of everything and everyone. In fact, with Pisces, spirit becomes the driver of our material world.

Imagine, for example, a digital radio. Without being plugged in to the wall to receive electricity, it is nothing but its parts—plastic, wire, and rubber. As soon as it is plugged in, however, it comes to life with songs, speeches, and as many sounds as you can find on its stations. Electricity, in this example, is the radio's *élan vital*, vital principle, source of life. It is not the songs or speeches it spews forth—nor the thoughts or emotions behind them—but their animating force. Such is spirit for your human body.

It is difficult to define something as qualitative as spirit, which is why it goes by many names (such as God, Yahweh, Source, the Light, energy, *prana*). Despite it being an essence that infuses everyone and everything, you cannot directly see, smell, or otherwise viscerally sense it. And so there is not enough agreement on what it means to give spirit the objectivity that the Western world requires for validation (note, though, that plenty of other belief systems are in full acceptance of what spirit is and represents). Thus, *spirit* means different things to different people, since one's experience with it is primarily subjective—residing in the realm of insights, instincts, and impressions versus linear, labeled thought.

Spirit is a shape-shifter that truly resides everywhere and in everything—from worldly wares like tables and chairs, to archetypes such as love and compassion. Unconditional love and compassion are forms of energy that, of all the zodiac signs, Pisces in particular is here to ground on planet Earth. So you must find practical ways to ground her otherwise lofty ideals. Typically, Pisces energy gravitates toward music, photography, art, and other creative media as a way to communicate spirit through form. But all types of daily choices—choosing sustainably raised food, buying ecologically sound cleaning products, volunteering for charities that help those in need—can also reflect Pisces's ideals. She shares the concept of service with Virgo, although Pisces serves from compassion rather than a sense of responsibility. She brings her elevated spirit to all because she sees spirit reflected in all.

But spirit needs form to bring it to life. That is why the Pisces Nobel laureate Albert Einstein was not renowned for just sitting and receiving brilliant insights that remained captive inside him but for turning his understandings into mathematical equations and then transferring those formulas onto chalkboards around the globe. Just like fellow Pisces Galileo Galilei gave the theory of heliocentrism tangible support through the astronomical observations he made and recorded from the telescope he invented. Numbers, chalkboards, pens, paper, telescopes . . . there are many ways to make the intangible tangible. Which is not to negate the existence of matter itself! Neither spirit nor matter is supreme—both require the other for completeness. And that's the whole point. Spirit moves matter just as matter moves spirit. How you view it is simply a matter (pun intended) of perspective—especially given that matter is really just one, dense form of energy.

In parts of Southeast Asia, like Bali, there is no word for *art* because every offering and act made is considered art—a gesture of spirit moving through matter.

As far as the Fish is concerned, however, matter acts as a container for spirit. Spirit is the clean, pure water that can serve any number of purposes depending on whether it is poured into a vase, run through a hydroelectric plant, or seeped through a cloth. There is no right or wrong type of container, simply the one that best serves Pisces's particular purpose. So it is for you to consider how your matter can serve your inner Pisces's purpose, an energy that typically finds itself at home in the arts world, using hands to draw, body to dance, eyes to photograph, and ears to compose what imagination and intuition understand.

Spirit imbuing different aspects of the arts is what has allowed so much art to successfully live hundreds of years. Pieces such as *Dance at Le Moulin de la Galette* by Pierre-Auguste Renoir; *Composition with Yellow, Blue, and Red* by Piet Mondrian; *Revolutionary Étude* by Frédéric Chopin; and *The Four Seasons* by Antonio Vivaldi are known around the globe because their Pisces creators invoked universal truths through art and music. Words cannot always fit such a large bill! And it is because spirit's message is universal in nature that words are not necessarily needed. We are able to understand expression of spirit in many forms, from art's canvas to the body's movements to emotion's tears; words, after all, are only one form of container.

Lessons

Forget about which shoe provides the perfect fit; every Pisces is really searching for how to allow her open, sensitive, watery nature to flow into our angular, mind-over-matter civilization. The Fish's energy barely has its own concrete shape, let alone the ones strongly encouraged by society. And yet, intangible energy needs to take form in a tangible world. So this sign's energy is here to figure out how her own shape takes root upon this Earth, how she can infuse her gifts throughout Earth's matter in order to help others do the same. Ultimately, grounding asserts your right to be, and your right to be here now. As in who you are, how you are, and where you are in your life at any given point in time. It is free of expectations from your parents, your job, your school—and even yourself. Being grounded in yourself means that there is nothing more that you need to do than to just be you, in your entirety—body and soul, matter and spirit.

If you are successful in this mission, you become a shining example of an enlightened being. Of an individual living her Pisces spirit through matter right here on Earth. Of course, easier said than done! For our modern world is matter-centric and even the simple word *spirit* is enough to close many eyes and minds. Funnily enough, the reverse prejudice might occur if you glom on to your Pisces's spiritual nature and eschew density of form. In this case, you will refuse to merge the two, and you run the risk of becoming ascetic. (This asceticism—and its resulting scarcity and austerity—is reflected in Pisces's season of birth, when winter is still ravaging the earth and the seeds of spring have yet to sprout.) Effectively, you will give up the good and bad wonders of the material world for what you perceive is a higher cause.

Another way of eschewing the material for the spiritual is by means of continual escapism, whether through delusions or drugs. In this scenario, you refuse to create the structure necessary to ground your Pisces spirit. When your spiritual circuitry runs wild with no container to be effectively channeled into and through, you start living apart from real life, which inevitably presents greater suffering than the spirit world. In this scenario, spirit and matter lack integration. And you then live life on this planet preferring to feel as if you were on another. Either way, if your Fish has no ground, it is possible that you have not yet found your true path in life.

Physical manifestations of an ungrounded Pisces energy may include:

* ★ High arches
* ★ Hypermobile feet
* ★ Frequent inversion of foot when walking (foot rolls under ankle, with sole pointing inward)
* ★ Inability to fully and stably plant foot on ground when standing or walking
* ★ Stubbed toes
* ★ Other: Growths (e.g., plantar warts, corns, calluses, bunions), joint degeneration

In contrast to remaining largely ensconced in the world of spirit, the other way unbalanced Fish energy might muck up your path is by being too grounded or incorrectly grounded. If you are too grounded, you might be spending more time than is good for you engaged in matters of body and mind while negating spirit; in so doing, you may be cultivating a connection with the material world that is closer than what is natural for you (unlike, for instance, the Taurus Bull who is all about earth and it is all she can do to lift her head to the heavens). Despite a highly sensitive nature, you might even shun all activities, books, talks, or ideas considered spiritual or fringe in order to not confront this Piscean aspect of yourself. This scenario is akin to forcing a whirling circle into a square hole. Or, while spirituality might be infused into your life, you may be grounding inappropriately through the wrong job, parental expectations, forced relationships, or the like. In both of these scenarios, incorrect grounding is occurring and your Fish feet will feel the resulting density of it.

Physical manifestations of an overly grounded Pisces nature may include:

* ★ The sensation of "heavy" or cement feet
* ★ Flat feet
* ★ Decreased range of mobility of ankles, feet, or toes
* ★ Burning on sole of foot

★ Pain or inflammation, typically on sole
★ Stubbed toes
★ Easily fatigued feet
★ Other: Growths (e.g., plantar warts, corns, calluses, bunions), joint degeneration

How well do your feet allow you to ground? Whether they feel ungrounded, overly grounded, or somewhere in between, the key is listening to your body and giving it what it needs. To stretch tight feet or strengthen weak ones, awaken your inner Pisces with the questions and exercises that follow.

Your Body and the Stars

The following will serve as your personal guide to embodying the Pisces stars. Use them to further integrate spirit into matter.

Questions

★ When you consider the various aspects of your life—from your role as parent to partner to employee and beyond—do you feel that, together, they form an integrated whole? Or do you feel that you are living as a series of disconnected parts?
★ What is your definition of *spirit*? What role does it play in your life?
★ What role would you like spirit to play in your life? What forms can you give it to make it part of your twenty-four-hour-a-day reality?
★ Do you feel that you are driven by your connection to the material world or the spiritual one? How would your life look and feel if the tables were turned?
★ What elements in your life make you feel less grounded? More grounded?
★ How would you qualitatively describe your feet (for example, cement-like, supple, achy, shaky, grounded)?

Exercises

Hand-to-Foot Pose: To Invoke Your Inner Zodiac

While it has no real beginning or end, the zodiac starts its cycle with Aries, the seed of new life that arrives in the spring. Its individuation into form begins a process that—eleven signs later—ends with the de-individuation of Pisces from self into spirit, only to find a new form with Aries again! It is a human journey that can be experienced within one lifetime (or many), through a confluence of body, mind, emotions, and spirit. Use this pose to create your own zodiac cycle by forming a physical one, and in so doing bringing your Aries head to your Pisces feet.

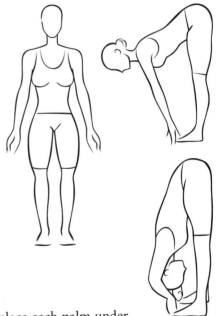

1. Start by standing upright with feet hip distance apart and arms hanging by your sides.
2. Inhale and, on the exhale, begin to roll down toward the ground, vertebra by vertebra. Your head will start the descent, followed by your neck, shoulders, torso, etc.
3. As you roll down, allow your arms to descend, catching your big toes with the thumb, second, and third fingers of each hand. If need be, bend your knees to make this connection possible.
4. Inhale and look up, straightening your back as much as possible.
5. Exhale and relax into the forward fold. Allow your head and neck to dangle. Remain here for five long, deep breaths.
6. To exit, return to the standing position by rolling up the way you came—vertebra by vertebra.

In this pose, the more advanced practitioner may place each palm under each sole of the foot to fully close the circuit. Less advanced practitioners may bring their hands to rest upon their shins.

Stomping: For Grounding

When you feel grounded, you feel more solid, stable, balanced, and supported. As if excess charge was removed from your day and you could breathe easily. Think about the last time you spent fifteen minutes frolicking barefoot on the grass to elicit the sensation. It turns out that one of the reasons you feel grounded when in contact with the ground is because earth literally acts as a ground—an object that transfers or receives electrons from another object (like your body) in order to neutralize it. Need a better reason to ground?! If so, see the Walk Barefoot exercise below. Otherwise, practice grounding (ideally outside and barefoot) with these simple stomps.

1. Stand upright, with bare feet shoulder distance apart and hands on your waist.
2. Bend your knees, shift your weight onto your left foot, lift your right foot as high as comfortably possible, and stomp it back down. Allow your foot to land flat and forcefully, as if you were pounding dough into the earth. Keep your body weight low, with knees bent. If it feels natural to release sound as you stomp, go for it!
3. When your right foot feels solidly planted, shift your weight onto it, raise your left one off the ground, and stomp it down.
4. Continue alternating sides for thirty seconds to one minute.

Stomping is a movement you have engaged in since you were a child, so you don't have to worry too much about form with this exercise (just keep an eye on how your knees handle your heft). The main focus should be on the solid, intentional connection you are forging with the earth, along with the myriad benefits you receive as a result.

Self Foot Massage: To Open into Spirit

Recall how the sign of Pisces incorporates all of the other signs into its one? The same is true for its physical counterpart, the foot. According to the field of reflexology, areas on each foot represent and connect to other areas of the body. So massaging the base of your arches is beneficial for your digestive organs as well. While ancient cultures in Egypt or China may have practiced similar techniques, reflexology was introduced to the United States by a physical therapist and medical doctor at the turn of the twentieth century. Since then, many individuals have found relief through reflexology—in fact, even a simple foot rub can often do wonders for foot pain. See for yourself, and practice the open-minded nature of the Pisces. You might not be able to practice actual reflexology on yourself at home, but this massage is a start to open you up to the wonders of your feet, new ways of healing, and from there—who knows?

1. Sit on a chair with your right leg crossed on top of the left, with the right ankle resting on top of the left thigh.
2. Hold the toes of your right foot with your right hand, and stabilize the heel with your left hand. With your right hand, gently extend the ankle and press back the toes for ten seconds. You should feel a stretch in the sole of the foot (along the plantar fascia).
3. Relax the foot for ten seconds. Repeat a total of ten times.
4. Add a massage: On the last repetition, hold your toes back, then use your left thumb to massage the sole of your foot, drawing lines from its ball to the heel. Start with the line formed by your inner arch, then move to the line on the inside of the foot, and then massage the line along the outer arch. Press as firmly as feels comfortable.
5. Repeat three times, and then switch feet.

Add in extra foot nourishment with essential oils as you massage your feet. Vetiver is one oil gifted at invoking the intuitive, spiritual aspects of Pisces's nature.

Word to the wise: Depending on the condition of your feet, they might feel sore after the first couple of times you massage them. If this is the case, your foot may just need a few days to become accustomed to the stretching and massaging, which helps mitigate muscular adhesions. The sensation should move from *ehhh* to *ahhh* shortly.

Seated Foot Stretch: To Shape Your Matter

Imagine a sculptor with a mound of clay. To her, any shape is possible. She transmits her vision through her hands and into the amorphous lump, ultimately manifesting whatever she wants to create, whether it's a coffee mug or a statue of a hug. While your physical form imposes greater limits than clay, for the most part you can also mold yourself in many different ways. To each their own: due to the angular orientation of your joints, along with the intrinsic flexibility of your ligaments, you will experience different limits and ranges of motion than everyone else. For this reason, some individuals may be born—or become—flexible enough to perform acrobatics while others, no matter how much they stretch, will not. The ideal way for your body to move is the ideal way your body can move.

You can decide how you want your feet to feel—healthy, open, breathing freely? What do you want them to do—run well, stand *en pointe*, maintain your balance? It is your choice. You get to infuse what you want and need in the reality literally at your feet. Your body is your structure—use this exercise to reintroduce yourself to it so that you may begin to shape it, lest it be shaped for you. For this exercise, you will need a resistance band. If you do not have one, you can approximate the band with a towel.

1. Sit on the floor with your legs elongated in front of you. You should be sitting on top of a neutral pelvis—please bend your knees if needed to sit properly upright and not cave in your lower back. Keep thighs, legs, and feet parallel to each other.
2. Hold both sides of the band in your right hand and wrap the band around the ball of your right foot, so that your toes are covered.
3. Slowly point your right toes—followed by your foot and ankle—toward the floor.
4. Extend them back toward you. Move slowly to feel the resistance as well as the articulation through each part of your toes, foot, and ankle.
5. Repeat five times, making sure that your torso remains straight while your feet are working.
6. With your foot still in the band, make five slow circles to the right and five to the left.
7. Change sides and repeat.

For more resistance, shorten the length of band. For less, lengthen it.

Walk Barefoot: For Integration

Right now, one or both of your feet are likely resting on the earth. The earth does a lot for us—it provides food and water and a terrain for walking, sitting, and building as well as natural and fulfilling energy. Earth's energy is an important part of feeling healthy and a reason why—in our cement-laden, industrialized society—you may not. Many health benefits may be derived from integrating your matter with the energy of the earth, from better balance, to a connection with nature, to improved foot health and strength. But to do this, you need to remove your shoes, socks, and other buffers that prevent you from connecting directly with the earth. Connect by walking barefoot on it—whether it is dirt or sand or grass—as frequently as possible, even if only for twenty seconds (but ideally for twenty minutes daily). This bare-foot adventure allows your feet to function free from interference like shoes. For an added bonus, walk in, near, or along water. Pisces is a water sign, and water is vital to the Fish at many levels, acting to calm, revive, and fulfill her.

Loving Meditation: To Cultivate Love and Compassion

It is impossible to write about Pisces without mentioning two characteristics that run deep within—a deep love of humanity and compassion that knows no bounds. As archetypes, love and compassion occupy the realm of spirit, and so it is of utmost importance that the Fish learn how to manifest these qualities into her physical form. Into the way she speaks, eats, relates, behaves, and moves. Of course, the first step is to get in touch with love and compassion, not through the understanding of the mind but by the knowing of the heart. Give it a try—you might be pleasantly surprised to learn how a five-minute meditation a day goes a long way.

1. Find a comfortable seat on the floor, sitting cross-legged upon a cushion, pillow, or block if needed (if cross-legged is not possible, find an easeful position sitting upright on a floor; if this position is not possible, sit on a chair).
2. Choose a space and time free from interruption. Turn off your phone ringer and set an alarm to alert you when this five-minute meditation is over.
3. Rest your palms facing up on your thighs, a posture of reception.
4. Allow your left hand to represent love and your right hand to represent compassion. Invoke the sensations by recalling prior situations in which you felt them.
5. Close your eyes and focus on your left hand in your mind's eye, invoking the thought and feeling of loving.
6. Now focus on your right hand in your mind's eye, invoking the thought and feeling of compassion. For help in this endeavor, recall a person, place, or thing that elicits the sensation.
7. Imagine a golden circle that connects your two hands.
8. Now, as you return your focus to love, trace a path along the top of the circle to bring you to compassion, and once at compassion, keep following the circle around the bottom back to love. With your eyes shut, keep tracing this circle between love and compassion, feeling one merge into the other.
9. After your alarm sounds, stay seated with eyes closed and pause for a moment. Reflect on the experience before you resume your day.

If five minutes seems daunting to you, feel free to practice this meditation in any lesser time interval that seems doable. The most important part of any meditation is simply showing up to do it. With practice, the length of your meditation will naturally increase over time.

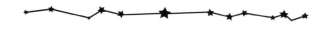

Summary

★ Your feet are the regions related to Pisces. Featuring an intricate interplay of bones, your feet allow the rest of you to interface—however you wish—with the ground below.

★ Pisces is the twelfth and final sign of the zodiac cycle. Its energy acknowledges the entire continuum of who you are from matter to spirit, and it asks that you integrate them in your life.

★ If your fluid Pisces nature becomes either too grounded or is not grounded enough, your feet might experience different symptoms (e.g., burning, heaviness).

★ Embrace your inner Pisces through questions, exercises, and activities that focus on your feet. Use them to remember that you are so much more than flesh and bones; you are walking, talking heaven on earth.

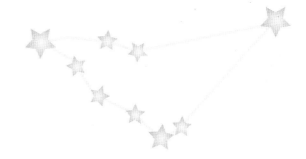

Conclusion

The main theme underlying this book-cum-wellness guide is that you are more than meets the eye, that your body, while made of stardust at the physical level, also reflects the cosmos at the metaphysical one. And by honoring this matter-spirit connection, you function as an interconnected whole—the whole that you deserve to be and know you are.

To not only believe it but truly live it, however, requires you to walk the talk—or, rather, practice the suggested questions and exercises that accompany each chapter or do whatever custom routine you create for yourself. The point is to lift the story off the pages, out of your head, and give it the reality of form. Align yourself through all the choices you make in a day, so who you are isn't just something you know inside but a reality you expressly live. It's like the example in the preface: you can think all you want about buying a house, but until you start taking the necessary steps, your house will remain nothing more than a dream.

And we believe that your dreams can come true, plus other great desires that you didn't even know you had—but you'll never know unless you try. And that's part of what we hope this book has encouraged you to do—to try something new, to embrace a new way of learning who you are. We hope that you are inspired to confront your weaknesses and transform challenges into strengths in order to open to a whole new definition of wellness. When you do—when you open yourself in this one area of your life—that openness resonates throughout all the others. Just like when you cultivate the compassion of the Pisces through a foot exercise, it doesn't last just five minutes but throughout the rest of the day, observable in subtle shifts like becoming more forgiving of yourself or more likely to open doors for others.

It is time to reconnect to our bodies and all they portend: from the grounding of our feet, to the love in our hearts, to the awareness of our heads. In other words: it is time to optimize your total health and well-being! Of the many ways to do this, this book offers you the wisdom of the stars as a means of holistic wellness—a practical and healing magic that allows you to tap into an ancient premise through the daily reality of your body. Because it shouldn't suffice for you to know the love that lives in your heart; you should relish in its expression by being able to feel it and live it through your movements, choice of words, posture, job, relationships, and so on. When this happens, it stops being just a concept and starts becoming real—this is why the questions, exercises, and activities in the book that help you call forth these otherwise intangible parts of yourself are so important. In practicing them regularly, you harness your own practical magic.

This book is about your daily routines and the practical magic that results from them. So put on your magician's hat! Continue to live through your body, the star that you are. Continually reach for the cosmos, inside and out, and remember that you reside in a universe that is constantly evolving—just as you are.

Thank you for taking this wellness journey from your body to the stars and back again. We hope that you enjoy living the book as much as we did creating it for you.

—Dr. Stephanie & Rebecca

Acknowledgments

To write a book about the body and stars requires seeing life as an interconnected whole. To that extent, we see all people and events in our lives as having helped this book take shape, and for that we are grateful. That said, there are a handful of individuals who played a direct role and to whom we offer direct gratitude: Robert Gottlieb and Mel Flashman at Trident Media Group for their foresight and faith; Emily Han, and Lindsay Easterbrooks-Brown, along with the whole team at Beyond Words Publishing for delivering our words into your hands with clarity and heart; all of the men and women who courageously volunteered their time, energy, and insights for our case studies (which ultimately didn't make it into the book but helped inform each chapter); and Dr. Roberta Rovner Pieczenik (Dr. Stephanie's mom), who has been editing Stephanie's papers since elementary school with love, devotion, and a keen eye toward excessive semicolon use. Finally, and with no less vim and vigor, we include heartfelt appreciation for all of our friends, family, and loved ones who have supported us along the way—you know who you are.

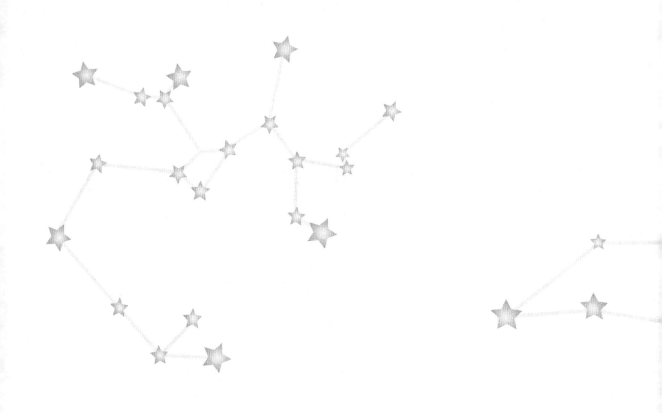

Appendix A:
Chart of Zodiac Signs and Physical Manifestations

The wisdom of each zodiac sign lives within you! And when you live in personal alignment with the wisdom, you feel balanced and well. Most of us, however, are still learning who we are and how best to live it, and at times we may feel un-well. Use any aches and pains as opportunities to learn more about yourself and how to care for yourself at all levels—body, mind, and spirit. What you perceive as wounds might actually be your greatest gifts.

Since this book features the body's musculoskeletal system, the manifestations included in the following table are primarily musculoskeletal as well (although some regions are more conducive to it than others). They are culled from the Lessons section of each chapter and represent what might arise if the energy of that sign is blocked from its full expression. As stated in the introduction, please use this table as a guide for further education and exploration of your body-mind-spirit connection (and not for diagnostic or predictive purposes).

Date*	Sun Sign	Body Regions	Physical Manifestations
Mar 21– Apr 19	Aries	Head	Headaches, migraines Irritated sinuses Head cold Stuffed or runny nose Eye infections Hair loss Ear infections Diminished hearing Tooth pain, infections, or grinding Tight jaw muscles Facial blemishes
Apr 20– May 20	Taurus	Neck	Tension or weakness, instability Stiffness or aching Restricted range of motion or hypermobility Crackling or crunching sensation Other: Cough, raw throat, throat infection, thyroid imbalance, soft or loud or unsteady voice
May 21– June 20	Gemini	Arms, forearms, hands	Shoulder, elbow, forearm, wrist, or hand pain Crackling or crunching sensation Weakness or tension Excessive knuckle popping Tight or winged shoulder blades Restricted movement or hypermobility Poor dexterity Weak grip or handshake

Date*	Sun Sign	Body Regions	Physical Manifestations
June 21–July 22	Cancer ♋	Chest	Tightness or aching Sunken or slumped kyphotic posture Shortness of breath Rib irritation, inflammation or injury Other: Respiratory dis-ease, esophageal dis-ease, excess phlegm, emotional eating, heartburn, breast lumps
July 23–Aug 22	Leo ♌	Heart, upper back	Puffed-out chest Slouched upper back or kyphotic posture Held or shallow breath Upper back tightness, tension, weakness, or fatigue Limited mobility Heart dis-ease
Aug 23–Sept 22	Virgo ♍	Abdomen	Rigid or weak core C-shaped, lordotic, or militaristic posture Shallow or held breath (versus belly breath) Other: Poor digestion, indigestion, food allergies, constipation, loose or irritable bowels, hernia, ulcers, disordered eating, hypochondriasis, obsessive behaviors

Date*	Sun Sign	Body Regions	Physical Manifestation
Sept 23– Oct 22	Libra	Lower back	Sore or tight muscles Muscle spasms Limited range of motion C-shaped, lordotic, or flat back posture Pain with sudden movements Pain or weakness with expenditure Symptoms of degeneration Other: Kidney or adrenal imbalance
Oct 23– Nov 21	Scorpio	Sacral center	Tight or weak muscles of the lower back, hamstrings, abdomen, gluteal region, or pelvic floor Ache or discomfort in the region of the lower back or gluteals Weakness or instability of pelvic region Restricted range of motion of the lower back or pelvis Hypermobility Fixed, non-neutral pelvis Excessive pelvic rotation, flare, or tilt Other: Menstrual cycle irregularity, urinary retention or incontinence or infection

Date*	Sun Sign	Body Regions	Physical Manifestation
Nov 22– Dec 21	Sagittarius	Hips, thighs	Tight or weak hip muscles Imbalanced hip muscles Fixed or excessive internal or external rotation of thighs Limited range of hip motion Hypermobility Iliotibial band tightness Non-neutral pelvic position Pain felt at or around the joint(s) Pinched nerve in the gluteal region and/or thigh Other: Over-indulgence in food or drink, liver imbalance
Dec 22– Jan 19	Capricorn	Knees	Tight or weak muscles and tendons surrounding the joint Achy pain or discomfort when moving or sitting Restricted or rigid range of motion Hyperextension Buckling or locking Crackling or crunching sensation or sound Excess fluid Shin splints Poor alignment

Date*	Sun Sign	Body Regions	Physical Manifestation
Jan 20– Feb 18	Aquarius	Ankles	Sensation of weakness or instability Rigidness or hypermobility Swelling Crackling feeling or sound Snapping sensation Instability of the joint Inversion of foot when walking Tight calf muscles Cramps or charley horse
Feb 19– Mar 20	Pisces	Feet	Hypermobility Inversion of foot when walking High or flat arches Unable to fully plant feet on ground Stubbing toes Heavy Burning sensation Painful sole Decreased range of motion Growths (e.g., corns, calluses) Degeneration

*Note

Keep in mind that you may see different dates in different charts. That is because of the precession of the equinox, which is the slow, backward motion that the Earth makes every seventy-two years, during which time the position of the stars changes by one degree.

Appendix B:
Body-of-the-Stars Scan

This full-body scan may be used:

★ To reconnect with your physical form and sense any blocks that may be obscuring the connection
★ To unite your body with its starry birthright and greater whole
★ For a meditative and relaxing experience
★ To establish a regular practice of self-care based on your zodiac needs

To begin, find a quiet spot to perform this exercise. It may take about five minutes, but you may extend it for as long as you like. On the floor or mat, enter into the yoga corpse pose by lying on your back with arms and legs extended, palms facing up, and eyes closed. Use props, as necessary, to make yourself comfortable. Starting with your focus on the head and ending at the feet, internally repeat the following phrases, taking a relaxed breath between each one:

★ I am Aries. I am my head. I am whole.

★ I am Taurus. I am my neck. I am whole.

★ I am Gemini. I am my arms, forearms, and hands. I am whole.

★ I am Cancer. I am my chest. I am whole.

★ I am Leo. I am my upper back and heart. I am whole.

★ I am Virgo. I am my abdomen. I am whole.

★ I am Libra. I am my lower back. I am whole.

★ I am Scorpio. I am my sacral center. I am whole.

★ I am Sagittarius. I am my hips and thighs. I am whole.

★ I am Capricorn. I am my knees. I am whole.

★ I am Aquarius. I am my ankles. I am whole.

★ I am Pisces. I am my feet. I am whole.

★ I accept the parts of my whole. I give gratitude to my whole. I relax into my whole.

Following the repetition, spend as long as you like in corpse pose, lying flat on the floor with your legs and arms elongated and relaxed.

Appendix C:
Your Body's Skeletal Structures and Regions

Skeletal Structure

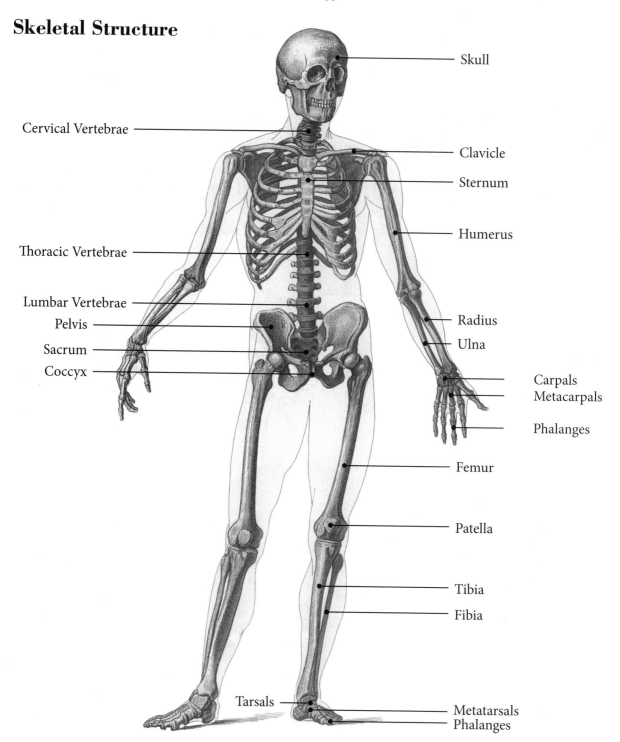

Skull

Cervical Vertebrae

Clavicle

Sternum

Humerus

Thoracic Vertebrae

Lumbar Vertebrae

Radius

Pelvis

Ulna

Sacrum

Coccyx

Carpals
Metacarpals

Phalanges

Femur

Patella

Tibia

Fibia

Tarsals

Metatarsals
Phalanges